Independent CPHON Study Guide 2027-2028:

600 Realistic Questions with Detailed Rationales Covering All Domains for the ONCC Certified Pediatric Hematology Oncology Nurse Exam

Caldwell Abiodun

📚 STUDY GUIDE BONUS MATERIAL

🎧 Full Audio Edition

Access the complete book in audio format
Ideal for learning during travel, workouts, or downtime
Stay productive even when you're not in the mood to read

📱 Digital Flashcards

Fast and effective revision tool
Strengthen memory of important concepts
Study anytime, wherever you are

⚡ Quick & Easy Access

No sign-up needed
Compatible with all devices
Smooth and instant usability

📍 ***Access all bonus content on Page 15***

Author Introduction

Pediatric hematology and oncology nursing is a highly specialized field dedicated to the care of children, adolescents, and families affected by cancer and blood disorders. The CPHON exam reflects the advanced knowledge, clinical judgment, and professional standards required to support safe, compassionate, and evidence-informed nursing care in this complex practice area.

The author of this study guide approaches CPHON exam preparation with a structured and clinically focused methodology designed to support meaningful understanding rather than simple recall. The development of this material reflects systematic analysis of the exam's professional content areas, including pediatric oncology and hematology concepts, treatment modalities, symptom management, supportive care, psychosocial considerations, patient and family education, ethical practice, and safety principles. Each section has been organized to reinforce the applied reasoning skills needed to evaluate patient needs, recognize complications, interpret clinical priorities, and connect nursing interventions to appropriate standards of care.

This guide emphasizes accuracy, clarity, and practical relevance throughout its instructional design. The author's approach incorporates careful review of domain expectations, current nursing terminology, common clinical scenarios, and the types of decision-making patterns that candidates are expected to demonstrate in certification-level assessment. Content has been shaped through editorial review and quality assurance practices intended to ensure consistency, readability, and professional usefulness for nurses preparing to validate specialized competency in pediatric hematology and oncology nursing.

Particular attention has been given to presenting complex clinical topics in a clear and organized manner while preserving the seriousness and depth of the specialty. The material supports candidates in strengthening both foundational knowledge and higher-level clinical reasoning, including prioritization, risk recognition, patient-centered communication, and safe care planning.

This study guide is designed as an independent educational resource for CPHON exam preparation. It reflects a commitment to professional advancement, nursing excellence, and the continued development of knowledgeable clinicians prepared to serve pediatric patients and families with skill, confidence, and compassion.

Table of Content

The information contained in this publication is provided for educational and informational purposes only. While every effort has been made to ensure the accuracy and reliability of the content at the time of publication, the author and contributing team make no representations or warranties regarding completeness, accuracy, or suitability for any specific purpose. Clinical guidelines, standards of care, and examination content may change over time. Readers are encouraged to consult current professional resources and institutional policies when applying any information in practice settings.

This publication is not affiliated with, endorsed by, or sponsored by any certifying body, professional organization, or examination board. All referenced trademarks, service marks, and certification marks are the property of their respective owners and are used strictly for identification purposes.

The publisher and contributors disclaim any liability for any loss, injury, or damage arising from the use or misuse of the information presented herein. Use of this material constitutes acceptance of these terms.

Disclaimer

CPHON® is a registered certification mark of the Oncology Nursing Certification Corporation. This publication is an independent study tool and is not affiliated with or endorsed by ONCC®.

Chapter-1: Care Continuum

Transition of Care

Coordinated Primary Care

Primary care forms the foundation of pediatric oncology nursing, ensuring that early symptoms of hematologic or oncologic disease are recognized promptly. Coordination between general pediatric providers and specialty teams allows for timely diagnostic workups and referrals. The nurse bridges these systems through communication and care documentation, maintaining safety during the transition from community to tertiary settings. In this phase, patient education focuses on understanding the illness trajectory, medication adherence, and the importance of follow-up appointments. Ongoing communication with the primary care provider supports immunization updates, developmental assessments, and family wellness promotion. The nurse also ensures that psychosocial support begins early, linking families to counseling or community resources as needed. Through collaboration and consistency, primary care provides the baseline stability required for comprehensive pediatric oncology management.

Continuity Across Care Levels

Children with hematologic or oncologic disorders move between hospitals, outpatient clinics, and home care. Each setting presents unique safety requirements, from infection control in the inpatient unit to medication adherence in the home environment. The nurse must adapt teaching strategies to each context while maintaining unified standards of care. Clear communication and shared documentation prevent fragmentation and duplication of services. Families receive coaching on managing central lines, nutrition, and symptom recognition. The goal is seamless care coordination that supports recovery, prevents complications, and sustains emotional well-being across transitions. The pediatric oncology nurse functions as a constant presence in this evolving continuum.

Discharge Planning and Preparation

Discharge planning begins at the time of admission and continues through every stage of therapy. The nurse leads the process by assessing family readiness, available resources, and potential barriers to home care. Education includes medication schedules, side effect management, infection prevention, and criteria for contacting the care team. The process integrates with school reintegration planning and community resource linkage. Discharge teaching is reinforced through demonstrations and return demonstrations to ensure comprehension. The nurse documents understanding and coordinates follow-up appointments to maintain continuity of care. This preparation ensures families feel confident and supported when the child returns home.

Integration of Palliative Care

When disease progression limits curative options, the transition to palliative care becomes a crucial part of the continuum. The nurse provides emotional and clinical support to guide families through decision-making and symptom management. Care shifts toward comfort, dignity, and family-centered priorities. Palliative interventions address physical symptoms such as pain and nausea, while also supporting emotional and spiritual needs. Collaboration with social workers, psychologists, and chaplains helps maintain holistic care. The nurse advocates for open communication, ensuring that family values are respected in treatment decisions. This integration maintains quality of life for both the patient and family.

Communication and Care Handoffs

Effective communication between healthcare teams prevents errors and promotes safe transitions. The nurse uses structured handoff tools to convey treatment progress, complications, and ongoing needs. Families are included in discussions to verify understanding and participation. Documentation is clear, timely, and accessible across all care platforms. Communication continues beyond discharge through telephone follow-ups or telehealth consultations. Consistency in language and shared decision-making fosters trust and transparency. These practices ensure that no aspect of care is lost during transitions.

Evaluation and Quality Improvement

Transition success is measured by stability, adherence, and family satisfaction. The nurse participates in reviewing outcome data such as readmission rates and post-discharge complications. Quality improvement initiatives may include standardized discharge checklists, electronic communication tools, and transition readiness assessments. Feedback from families informs future process refinements. Ongoing staff education ensures team alignment with national standards. Each evaluation cycle strengthens the safety and efficiency of pediatric oncology transitions. The goal is to sustain excellence across all phases of care delivery.

Health Promotion and Maintenance

Preventive Health and Screening

Health promotion begins with preventing infection, malnutrition, and treatment-related complications. Nurses perform routine screenings for developmental milestones, growth, and early signs of therapy toxicity. Preventive education includes hygiene, nutrition, and rest. The nurse works with families to minimize environmental exposures that compromise immunity. Immunization schedules are adapted based on immune status, ensuring safety and efficacy. Surveillance for secondary health issues such as hypertension or endocrine imbalance continues throughout and after therapy. Prevention remains a lifelong aspect of pediatric oncology care.

Family Education and Empowerment

Family education transforms caregivers into capable partners in care. Teaching emphasizes medication administration, recognizing early warning signs, and maintaining safe environments. Education is tailored to literacy levels and cultural contexts. Visual aids and demonstration models enhance comprehension. Empowered families are better able to advocate for their child's needs and collaborate with healthcare professionals. The nurse's role includes reinforcing information over time and evaluating understanding. Education becomes both a safety tool and a means of emotional reassurance.

Nutrition and Physical Activity

Nutrition supports immune function, wound healing, and energy balance during therapy. The nurse collaborates with dietitians to address caloric needs, taste changes, and treatment-induced nausea. Encouraging small, frequent meals and hydration helps reduce fatigue and malnutrition. As recovery progresses, moderate physical activity promotes endurance and psychological well-being. Nurses teach families how to balance rest and movement safely. Guidance extends to managing cachexia and appetite suppression associated with chemotherapy. Holistic attention to nutrition and activity strengthens overall resilience.

Psychological and Emotional Wellness

Health promotion extends to mental health. The nurse screens for anxiety, depression, and coping difficulties in both child and family members. Open dialogue, active listening, and referral to counseling resources help address emotional stress. Nurses incorporate therapeutic play and age-appropriate discussions to support coping. Families are encouraged to maintain routines and celebrate small milestones. Emotional stability enhances compliance and improves recovery outcomes. A nurturing environment supports the child's overall healing process.

Environmental and Safety Management

Maintaining a safe environment is central to health promotion. Nurses educate caregivers about reducing infection risks, managing hazardous medications, and ensuring clean home conditions. Proper handling of chemotherapy waste and personal protective equipment is reinforced. Safety planning includes fire prevention, safe toy selection, and fall risk reduction. Environmental safety protects vulnerable immune systems and prevents secondary injuries. Home evaluations and community referrals strengthen sustainability. The nurse ensures all family members understand safety as a shared responsibility.

Monitoring for Late and Secondary Effects

Treatment can lead to long-term consequences such as cardiomyopathy, infertility, or learning challenges. Nurses coordinate follow-up assessments and ensure that families understand the purpose of long-term monitoring. Early identification allows for timely intervention and improved outcomes. Survivorship programs provide structured evaluation schedules and education. Nurses emphasize the importance of lifelong follow-up and documentation of past treatments. This proactive approach minimizes late morbidity. Health maintenance thus becomes a continuous process extending into adulthood.

Survivorship

Understanding Survivorship

Survivorship begins the day treatment starts and continues throughout life. It recognizes the medical and psychosocial challenges that follow recovery from pediatric cancer or blood disorders. Nurses provide education about long-term risks and encourage proactive health management. Survivorship care includes both surveillance for late effects and promotion of wellness behaviors. The nurse facilitates open communication between survivors, families, and multidisciplinary teams. Survivorship is not the end of care but a continuation of the healing journey.

Physical and Functional Recovery

Physical rehabilitation restores strength, mobility, and normal growth patterns after treatment. Nurses assess fatigue, neuropathy, and musculoskeletal weakness, providing strategies for gradual improvement. Collaboration with physiotherapists ensures safe and progressive exercise regimens. Regular assessments track recovery milestones such as endurance and flexibility. Attention to energy balance, nutrition, and hydration accelerates healing. The goal is to rebuild physical confidence and independence in daily activities.

Cognitive and Developmental Reintegration

Cognitive changes may arise from chemotherapy, radiation, or prolonged hospitalization. Nurses monitor for learning difficulties, concentration issues, and school reintegration challenges. Coordination with educators and psychologists ensures academic accommodations and developmental continuity. Guidance for parents focuses on recognizing subtle behavioral shifts that may indicate cognitive fatigue. Structured support helps the child regain confidence in learning and social interactions. Cognitive recovery is a critical measure of successful survivorship.

Emotional and Social Adaptation

Survivors and families often face anxiety about recurrence and identity changes post-treatment. Nurses encourage emotional expression and connect families with peer support programs. Reintegration into peer groups and normal activities rebuilds social stability. Adolescents benefit from counseling focused on body image, independence, and future planning. Families receive reassurance that emotional ups and downs are part of healing. The nurse serves as a consistent advocate for emotional resilience.

Long-Term Health Education

Education focuses on empowering survivors to manage their own health responsibly. Nurses teach self-assessment for unusual symptoms, adherence to medical follow-up, and lifestyle optimization. Survivors learn to communicate their medical history to future healthcare providers. Teaching emphasizes avoidance of tobacco, alcohol, and high-risk behaviors. Education also addresses reproductive health and fertility considerations. Knowledge becomes the survivor's lifelong tool for self-protection.

Transition to Adult Care

As survivors reach adolescence and adulthood, seamless transfer to adult healthcare providers becomes essential. Nurses prepare detailed treatment summaries and educate new providers on prior therapies and potential late effects. Families are guided to identify adult specialists familiar with survivorship care. The transition process empowers patients to manage appointments and medications independently. Emotional readiness is assessed to ensure confidence in self-advocacy. Successful transition maintains surveillance continuity and lifelong wellness support.

Chapter-2: Pediatric Hematology and Oncology Nursing Practice

Pediatric Cancers and Hematologic Disorders

Understanding Disease Presentation

Children with hematologic or oncologic disorders often present with symptoms that differ from adults, requiring a nuanced assessment approach. The pediatric nurse must recognize early warning signs such as fatigue, petechiae, bone pain, or persistent infections. Early detection depends on careful observation of subtle physical and behavioral changes reported by families. Understanding normal growth and development assists in identifying abnormal patterns suggestive of disease. Comprehensive assessment includes evaluation of nutritional status, immunologic function, and psychosocial indicators. The nurse synthesizes these findings to support timely diagnosis and referral. Early recognition directly influences prognosis and treatment outcomes.

Anatomy, Physiology, and Pathophysiology

A firm grasp of hematopoietic and oncologic physiology underpins safe and effective care. The nurse must understand how bone marrow dysfunction, genetic mutations, or immune dysregulation contribute to malignant transformation. In hematologic disorders such as sickle cell disease, pathophysiology includes altered erythrocyte morphology and impaired oxygen delivery. Oncologic conditions, including leukemias and solid tumors, result from uncontrolled cell proliferation and resistance to apoptosis. Nurses translate complex biological concepts into practical care strategies, such as monitoring lab results and interpreting treatment effects. Knowledge of organ systems most affected by therapy—liver, kidney, heart—guides targeted assessment. Pathophysiologic insight ensures individualized, safe, and precise nursing interventions.

Genetic and Genomic Considerations

Genomic research has transformed pediatric oncology, highlighting the role of chromosomal translocations and inherited mutations in disease development. Nurses explain genetic testing processes and implications to families in clear, compassionate language. Awareness of hereditary cancer syndromes assists in family risk counseling and surveillance recommendations. The nurse supports families during genomic result disclosure, addressing concerns about stigma and future fertility. Integration of genetics into nursing care helps tailor therapies such as targeted agents or immunotherapies. Continuous education ensures nurses remain informed on advances in molecular diagnostics. This understanding strengthens patient-centered care through precision medicine approaches.

Diagnostic Testing and Interpretation

Accurate diagnosis depends on laboratory and imaging evaluations. The nurse prepares children for procedures such as bone marrow aspiration, lumbar puncture, or central line insertion, using age-appropriate teaching and comfort techniques. Understanding diagnostic tests—complete blood counts, flow cytometry, cytogenetic panels—enables the nurse to interpret trends and report abnormalities promptly. Collaboration with the healthcare team ensures that findings are correlated with clinical presentation. Nurses also manage procedural anxiety through distraction, parental presence, and relaxation methods. Documentation of tolerance and response supports holistic care. Diagnostic proficiency enhances safety and confidence in clinical practice.

Staging, Prognosis, and Clinical Communication

Staging establishes disease extent and informs treatment decisions. The nurse must comprehend staging terminology for both hematologic malignancies and solid tumors, including cytogenetic risk stratification. Prognosis discussions are emotionally charged and require empathetic communication skills. Nurses support families during multidisciplinary meetings, helping them process information and set realistic expectations. Understanding prognostic indicators such as tumor histology or minimal residual disease helps nurses anticipate complications and provide individualized support. Transparent communication builds trust and fosters collaborative decision-making. The nurse's interpretive and emotional role is integral to maintaining family stability.

Holistic Family-Centered Assessment

Beyond physical symptoms, the nurse evaluates the family's emotional, financial, and social readiness to manage chronic illness. Assessment includes caregiver coping capacity, sibling understanding, and access to community support. Nurses employ culturally sensitive approaches that respect diverse family structures and belief systems. Holistic assessment guides referrals to social work, psychology, and educational support services. Recognizing caregiver burnout and anticipatory grief allows timely intervention. By treating the family as a unit of care, the nurse ensures that emotional resilience and comprehension accompany clinical progress. Holistic understanding forms the foundation for sustained healing.

Clinical Trials

Phases of Clinical Trials

Clinical trials drive innovation in pediatric hematology and oncology care. Nurses must understand the four major phases: safety evaluation, dosage determination, efficacy testing, and post-market surveillance. Each phase has unique ethical and procedural implications. The nurse educates families about trial goals, risks, and potential benefits, ensuring informed decision-making. Vigilant observation for adverse reactions maintains participant safety. Accurate documentation and adherence to protocols safeguard research integrity. The nurse's role extends beyond monitoring to advocacy, ensuring voluntary participation and comprehension throughout the trial process.

Informed Consent and Ethical Safeguards

Ethical practice requires that consent be fully informed, voluntary, and developmentally appropriate. Nurses explain complex information in accessible terms for both parents and adolescent patients. Consent discussions address confidentiality, withdrawal rights, and potential side effects. Cultural and linguistic barriers are identified and managed through interpreters and educational aids. The nurse acts as the family's advocate, verifying that consent is obtained without coercion or misunderstanding. Documentation reflects both comprehension and voluntary agreement. Ethical vigilance protects participant autonomy and preserves public trust in research.

Data Integrity and Reporting

Accurate and timely data recording is essential in clinical trials. Nurses maintain meticulous logs of medication administration, side effects, and patient responses. Adherence to Good Clinical Practice (GCP) guidelines ensures reproducibility and compliance. Deviations are reported immediately through established research channels. Data quality directly affects the credibility of study outcomes. The nurse collaborates with research coordinators and principal investigators to maintain regulatory standards. Precision and accountability safeguard the scientific value of pediatric oncology research.

Safety Monitoring and Adverse Event Management

Monitoring for toxicity and adverse reactions is a primary nursing responsibility. The nurse assesses laboratory parameters, observes clinical signs, and communicates concerns promptly. Emergency preparedness includes familiarity with study-specific management protocols. Early recognition of hypersensitivity, infection, or organ dysfunction minimizes risk. Nurses reinforce adherence to monitoring schedules and provide reassurance during testing. Their vigilance protects the patient while ensuring data reliability. Safety remains the defining principle of ethical research practice.

Education and Communication in Research Participation

Families require clear, consistent updates throughout the study period. The nurse explains procedures, timelines, and expected side effects in accessible language. Continuous dialogue reduces anxiety and promotes adherence. Written materials and visual tools enhance comprehension. The nurse bridges communication between investigators and participants, translating technical terminology into meaningful understanding. Open, empathetic communication ensures that research participation aligns with family values and expectations. Education sustains trust throughout the clinical trial journey.

Interdisciplinary Collaboration

Clinical trials require collaboration between physicians, pharmacists, laboratory staff, and nurses. The pediatric nurse coordinates medication preparation, verifies protocol accuracy, and ensures environmental safety during administration. Collaboration enhances precision and efficiency. Team debriefings support continuous quality improvement and safety validation. Interdisciplinary synergy reinforces shared accountability for ethical research conduct. The nurse's leadership within this team framework reflects professionalism and scientific integrity.

Professional Performance

Scope and Standards of Practice

Professional standards guide nursing performance within pediatric hematology and oncology. The nurse practices under defined scopes established by institutional policy and national guidelines. Adherence to these standards ensures accountability, patient safety, and ethical integrity. Ongoing professional development maintains competence in rapidly evolving clinical areas. Nurses apply critical thinking to adapt evidence-based guidelines to individual patient contexts. Maintaining scope alignment reinforces public trust in nursing practice.

Ethical and Legal Principles

Ethical decision-making in pediatric oncology often involves balancing beneficence, autonomy, and justice. Nurses confront dilemmas related to experimental treatments, end-of-life decisions, and resource allocation. Legal frameworks support patient rights and protect vulnerable populations. The nurse applies ethical reasoning models to guide communication and intervention. Documentation reflects transparency and adherence to ethical codes. Maintaining integrity within legal boundaries safeguards both patient welfare and professional credibility.

Patient and Family Education

Education remains a cornerstone of professional nursing performance. Nurses tailor teaching strategies to cultural backgrounds, literacy levels, and emotional states. Reinforcement through verbal explanation, demonstration, and written resources promotes understanding. Family participation strengthens adherence to complex treatment plans. Effective education fosters empowerment, confidence, and safety. Continuous evaluation ensures educational goals align with patient progress and comprehension.

Interdisciplinary Collaboration and Leadership

Pediatric oncology nursing thrives within multidisciplinary collaboration. Nurses communicate with physicians, pharmacists, therapists, and educators to coordinate comprehensive care. Leadership involves proactive problem-solving and advocacy for patient-centered priorities. The nurse models teamwork behaviors, mentors new staff, and promotes mutual respect across disciplines. Collaboration improves clinical efficiency and enhances family satisfaction. Leadership ensures care unity despite the complexity of treatment.

Regulatory and Safety Standards

Compliance with institutional, national, and international regulations ensures safe and ethical practice. Nurses maintain familiarity with chemotherapy handling protocols, radiation safety, and infection control measures. Accurate documentation and error reporting support transparency and continuous improvement. Adherence to safety regulations reduces occupational and patient risk. Regular audits and competency assessments validate practice quality. Regulatory compliance anchors professional accountability.

Commitment to Lifelong Learning

Professional excellence requires ongoing education and reflective practice. Nurses pursue certifications, workshops, and continuing education to maintain expertise. Participation in professional organizations promotes networking and knowledge exchange. Reflective journaling and peer discussions enhance self-awareness and critical thinking. Continuous learning ensures adaptation to evolving technologies and therapies. The commitment to lifelong growth defines professional identity and elevates care quality.

Access Audio file and Flashcards

Scan QR Code Below

Chapter-3: Treatment Modalities and Side Effects

Hematologic Treatment Approaches

Chemotherapy Principles

Chemotherapy remains central to the treatment of pediatric hematologic disorders. It involves the administration of cytotoxic agents that target rapidly dividing cells, requiring precise dosing and vigilant monitoring. Nurses must understand mechanisms of action, potential toxicities, and safe handling procedures to ensure optimal outcomes. Prior to administration, accurate body surface area calculations and double-checking by two qualified professionals reduce dosing errors. Anticipatory guidance prepares families for side effects such as nausea, alopecia, or myelosuppression. Nurses manage adverse effects with hydration, antiemetic therapy, and infection prevention strategies. Education on home safety for oral chemotherapy supports adherence and protects caregivers. Continuous assessment of response and toxicity ensures safe and effective therapy delivery.

Biotherapy and Immunotherapy

Biotherapy uses biological agents to enhance or restore the body's immune system in combating cancer and hematologic diseases. Nurses monitor for hypersensitivity reactions, cytokine release syndromes, and infusion-related side effects. Detailed premedication protocols and emergency readiness are critical to patient safety. Education focuses on helping families recognize early signs of immune-mediated reactions at home. Immunotherapies such as monoclonal antibodies and checkpoint inhibitors require understanding of specific target mechanisms and long-term monitoring for delayed toxicities. Nurses coordinate laboratory surveillance and communicate promptly with providers regarding abnormal findings. This approach exemplifies precision care in modern pediatric oncology.

Blood Product Therapy

Transfusion of red cells, platelets, or plasma products supports patients experiencing anemia, thrombocytopenia, or coagulopathy during therapy. The nurse's role includes verifying patient identity, product compatibility, and infusion rate. Vigilant observation for transfusion reactions—fever, hives, respiratory distress—ensures rapid intervention. Education for families covers recognition of delayed transfusion effects and the importance of follow-up laboratory evaluation. Safe handling, documentation, and adherence to institutional policies prevent complications. Maintaining sterility and monitoring vital signs enhance safety. Blood product therapy stabilizes hematologic parameters and supports ongoing treatment tolerance.

Hematopoietic Stem Cell Transplantation

Stem cell transplantation offers potential cure for high-risk hematologic malignancies and bone marrow failure syndromes. Nurses play key roles in pre-transplant conditioning, donor coordination, and post-transplant monitoring. Complications such as graft-versus-host disease and infection demand meticulous surveillance. Patient education addresses isolation precautions, medication adherence, and emotional coping during prolonged hospitalization. Post-discharge follow-up focuses on immunization schedules, nutritional support, and reintegration into school and community life. The nurse ensures consistency between inpatient and outpatient teams. Compassionate communication sustains family resilience during this complex process.

Surgical Interventions

Surgery may be required for biopsy, tumor resection, or central line placement. Nurses prepare patients through preoperative teaching that includes fasting guidelines, anesthesia expectations, and postoperative pain control. Post-surgical care emphasizes wound monitoring, infection prevention, and early mobilization. Nurses collaborate with surgeons and physical therapists to optimize recovery. Emotional preparation for both patient and family reduces anxiety. Clear communication about expected outcomes builds trust. The nurse's vigilance during perioperative phases ensures safety and comfort.

Coagulation Therapy and Supportive Agents

Children with hematologic disorders such as hemophilia or disseminated intravascular coagulation require targeted coagulation management. Nurses administer factor replacement therapy, antifibrinolytics, and monitor for bleeding complications. Education focuses on avoiding trauma and recognizing early signs of hemorrhage. Coordination with hematology specialists ensures appropriate factor dosing and documentation. Home therapy programs emphasize independence and safety. Nurses advocate for school accommodations and emergency action plans. Effective coagulation management supports both physical safety and quality of life.

Oncologic Treatment Approaches

Chemotherapy in Solid Tumors

Chemotherapy for solid tumors often involves combination regimens targeting different cellular pathways. The nurse's responsibility includes ensuring drug compatibility, monitoring for extravasation, and managing cumulative organ toxicity. Patient and family education addresses potential late effects such as infertility or hearing loss. Nurses monitor renal and hepatic function, adjusting hydration protocols as necessary. Managing nausea and mucositis enhances comfort and nutritional intake. Long-term follow-up ensures that growth and development continue post-therapy. Continuous education empowers families to manage care safely at home.

Biotherapy in Oncology

Biologic agents in oncology, including cytokines, monoclonal antibodies, and vaccines, enhance immune-mediated tumor control. Nurses must anticipate and manage immune-related adverse events such as rash, colitis, or endocrinopathy. Ongoing assessment of inflammatory markers and organ function is vital. Families receive education about immune response expectations and self-monitoring for late toxicities. The nurse fosters understanding of the difference between immune activation symptoms and infection. Patient reassurance and symptom tracking promote adherence. This therapy represents a bridge between oncology and immunology, demanding high-level nursing competence.

Cellular Therapy and CAR-T Cell Treatment

Chimeric antigen receptor T-cell therapy (CAR-T) exemplifies cutting-edge personalized oncology care. Nurses provide pre-treatment education about lymphodepleting chemotherapy, infusion processes, and potential complications. Vigilant monitoring for cytokine release syndrome and neurotoxicity is essential during and after infusion. Interventions may include antipyretics, corticosteroids, or intensive care support. Families are counseled on early symptom recognition and emergency contacts after discharge. Emotional support during waiting periods for therapeutic effect reduces anxiety. Nurses contribute to research registries and long-term data collection, ensuring safety and advancement of this emerging therapy.

Radiation Therapy

Radiation therapy requires coordination of complex technical and safety measures. Nurses educate families about immobilization devices, potential side effects, and skin care during treatment. Assessment focuses on local reactions, fatigue, and mucosal irritation. The nurse collaborates with radiation therapists to ensure proper shielding and positioning. Education includes avoidance of irritants and maintenance of nutrition and hydration. Psychosocial preparation, particularly for younger children, minimizes fear of equipment and isolation. Post-treatment monitoring addresses delayed growth or endocrine dysfunction. Nursing vigilance sustains both safety and emotional comfort throughout the process.

Surgical Oncology and Postoperative Care

Surgery for tumor removal demands meticulous pre- and postoperative care. Nurses ensure informed consent, baseline laboratory testing, and family readiness before surgery. After surgery, pain control, wound integrity, and fluid balance become primary priorities. The nurse monitors for complications such as bleeding, infection, or impaired mobility. Emotional support for body image concerns, particularly following disfiguring procedures, is essential. Collaboration with rehabilitation specialists aids physical recovery and adaptation. Ongoing communication with the multidisciplinary team ensures comprehensive postoperative management.

Comprehensive Side Effect Management

Every treatment modality introduces side effects requiring proactive nursing interventions. Common toxicities include nausea, mucositis, alopecia, neuropathy, and fatigue. Nurses provide anticipatory guidance, pharmacologic management, and supportive counseling. Hydration, dietary modification, and infection prevention are reinforced. Emotional support and body image counseling improve coping and adherence. Monitoring for late effects such as cardiomyopathy or renal dysfunction ensures ongoing vigilance. Comprehensive side effect management underscores the nurse's role as both clinician and advocate for holistic well-being.

Integrative Support and Coordination

Medication Safety and Administration Standards

Safe medication administration relies on precision, verification, and teamwork. Nurses adhere to double-check policies, maintain sterile technique, and confirm dosing based on verified body metrics. Understanding drug pharmacokinetics and potential interactions prevents complications. Nurses advocate for system safeguards such as barcode scanning and computerized order entry. Continuous education on new agents maintains safety awareness. Families are educated about storage, handling, and disposal of hazardous drugs at home. Safe practice protects both patients and healthcare professionals.

Psychosocial Support During Treatment

The psychological toll of treatment demands structured emotional care. Nurses use active listening, play therapy, and counseling referrals to support children and families. Consistent communication reduces fear and uncertainty. Nurses encourage peer interaction in safe environments to prevent isolation. Recognizing caregiver fatigue leads to timely interventions. Integrating mental health care promotes adherence and resilience. Compassionate presence remains as vital as medical expertise in pediatric oncology.

Interdisciplinary Collaboration in Treatment Planning

Effective treatment depends on collaboration among oncologists, hematologists, nurses, dietitians, pharmacists, and therapists. The nurse coordinates communication, ensuring that families understand complex information. Team conferences align goals, prevent duplication, and streamline interventions. Shared decision-making enhances family confidence and satisfaction. Documentation reflects unified care planning. Interdisciplinary teamwork embodies the patient-centered philosophy of pediatric oncology.

Patient and Family Education

Continuous education supports treatment adherence and empowers families. Nurses use teach-back methods to verify understanding. Education covers drug purposes, side effects, and safety practices. Written schedules and symptom logs assist families in managing care at home. Education adapts to developmental levels, cultural contexts, and learning preferences. Empowered families actively participate in decision-making and daily care. Ongoing teaching ensures informed and safe participation in therapy.

Long-Term Monitoring and Survivorship Preparation

Monitoring continues long after active treatment concludes. Nurses track laboratory values, imaging results, and organ function to detect late effects early. Education about potential long-term complications prepares families for proactive health management. Survivorship planning includes lifestyle guidance, reproductive counseling, and vaccination updates. Coordination between oncology and primary care ensures continuity. Empowering survivors with health knowledge fosters lifelong vigilance and independence. This ongoing relationship symbolizes the enduring role of the pediatric oncology nurse.

Ethical Considerations in Treatment

Ethical decision-making permeates all treatment phases. Nurses balance the principles of beneficence, autonomy, and nonmaleficence in daily care. Conversations about experimental therapies, fertility preservation, or quality of life require sensitivity and honesty. Respect for cultural beliefs and family values guides ethical dialogue. Advocacy ensures that children's voices are considered in age-appropriate ways. The nurse upholds dignity and compassion regardless of prognosis. Ethical integrity anchors every intervention and defines professional excellence.

Chapter-4: Symptom Management and Supportive Care

System-Specific Effects

Neurological Complications

Neurological complications in pediatric oncology include seizures, neuropathies, and cognitive changes related to disease or therapy. Nurses assess for early signs such as headache, vision disturbances, altered reflexes, or gait instability. Continuous monitoring allows for rapid intervention, preventing irreversible damage. Nursing care involves maintaining safety, ensuring seizure precautions, and coordinating neuroimaging or consultations when indicated. Supportive strategies include energy conservation, structured routines, and cognitive rehabilitation exercises. Education for families emphasizes medication adherence and environmental safety to reduce risk of injury. Emotional support for families coping with neurological changes strengthens adaptation and understanding. Nurses also advocate for educational accommodations when cognitive impairment affects learning. A holistic approach ensures both physical safety and emotional comfort throughout recovery.

Respiratory and Cardiovascular Effects

Respiratory and cardiovascular complications often result from infection, fluid overload, or cardiotoxic treatments. Nurses perform frequent assessments of breathing patterns, oxygen saturation, and cardiac rhythm. Early detection of dyspnea or tachycardia prompts timely interventions such as oxygen therapy or diuretics. Collaboration with respiratory therapists supports ventilatory management and pulmonary hygiene. Education focuses on infection prevention, hydration balance, and recognizing warning signs at home. Cardiac monitoring is essential during administration of anthracyclines or radiation near the chest. Emotional reassurance and age-appropriate explanations help alleviate fear of medical devices and procedures. Nurses advocate for long-term follow-up with cardiology for patients at risk of late cardiac effects. This vigilance preserves cardiac and respiratory health across the treatment continuum.

Gastrointestinal and Nutritional Concerns

Chemotherapy and radiation frequently cause nausea, vomiting, mucositis, and diarrhea. Nurses administer antiemetic regimens and encourage small, frequent meals to maintain nutrition. Oral care protocols minimize mucosal injury and infection risk. Hydration is closely monitored to prevent electrolyte imbalance. Nutritional counseling supports caloric intake despite altered taste and appetite suppression. The nurse collaborates with dietitians to adjust textures and introduce nutrient-dense foods. Education for parents includes recognizing dehydration signs and maintaining hygiene during feeding. Emotional encouragement helps reduce mealtime stress. Attention to both physical and psychosocial aspects of eating preserves strength and recovery potential.

Renal and Endocrine Dysfunction

Certain chemotherapeutic agents and radiation therapies place the kidneys and endocrine glands at risk for long-term impairment. Nurses monitor urine output, laboratory values, and growth patterns to detect nephrotoxicity or hormonal imbalances early. Education emphasizes adequate fluid intake and avoidance of nephrotoxic substances. Collaboration with nephrologists and endocrinologists ensures specialized care when abnormalities arise. Hormonal monitoring includes assessment for delayed puberty, growth retardation, and thyroid dysfunction. Emotional support for adolescents coping with body image changes fosters confidence. Nurses guide families through management options, including hormone replacement or dietary adjustments. Ongoing evaluation ensures stable renal and metabolic function throughout and after therapy.

Hematologic and Immunologic Management

Cytopenias and immune suppression are common consequences of therapy. Nurses monitor complete blood counts and enforce infection prevention measures, including hand hygiene and isolation protocols when necessary. Education for families emphasizes avoiding crowds and reporting fevers promptly. Prophylactic medications such as growth factors and antibiotics are administered with strict adherence to guidelines. Nurses provide transfusion support as needed and assess for bleeding or bruising. Emotional support reduces anxiety related to frequent testing and hospitalizations. Reinforcing coping skills empowers children to participate in their care safely. Sustained vigilance preserves immune stability and minimizes complications.

Musculoskeletal and Integumentary Support

Therapy-related fatigue, steroid-induced weakness, and skin fragility require targeted nursing interventions. Nurses encourage gentle physical activity to prevent deconditioning and maintain mobility. Physical and occupational therapists collaborate to create individualized exercise plans. Skin care includes regular inspection for pressure injuries, rash, or infection. Topical treatments and protective dressings minimize discomfort and promote healing. Families learn positioning and mobility techniques to prevent strain and injury. Supportive footwear and adaptive devices enhance independence. Addressing physical and skin-related concerns restores confidence and reduces complications during therapy.

General Acute, Chronic, and Late Effects

Pain Management

Pain may arise from tumor pressure, procedures, or treatment toxicity. Nurses perform systematic assessments using age-appropriate pain scales and implement multimodal relief strategies. Pharmacologic management includes opioids, non-opioid analgesics, and adjuvant medications. Nonpharmacologic interventions such as relaxation, imagery, and play therapy enhance comfort. Continuous monitoring ensures balance between pain control and side effect minimization. Families receive education on dosing schedules and safe storage of medications. Empowering children to communicate pain levels improves accuracy and trust. Pain management extends to emotional distress, recognizing that anxiety often amplifies perceived discomfort. Compassionate attention to pain supports both healing and dignity.

Fatigue and Energy Conservation

Cancer-related fatigue affects physical activity, cognition, and mood. Nurses assess fatigue patterns and collaborate with families to balance rest and activity. Education emphasizes prioritizing essential tasks and maintaining nutrition and hydration. Encouragement of gentle exercise such as stretching or short walks helps sustain muscle tone. Sleep hygiene education promotes restorative rest. Emotional support reassures families that fatigue is a common and manageable symptom. Coordination with rehabilitation services helps optimize stamina. Recognizing fatigue as multifactorial guides comprehensive, compassionate care.

Sleep Disturbance and Circadian Disruption

Hospital routines, anxiety, and medication schedules frequently disrupt sleep patterns. Nurses promote consistent bedtime routines and quiet environments to encourage rest. Avoiding stimulants, minimizing nighttime interruptions, and using comfort objects can improve sleep quality. Education for parents emphasizes the value of maintaining sleep consistency even during hospitalization. Nurses evaluate for underlying causes such as pain or medication effects. Relaxation techniques and cognitive-behavioral approaches reduce insomnia. Adequate rest enhances immune recovery and emotional stability. Continuous assessment ensures individualized sleep support.

Mental Health and Emotional Resilience

Psychological symptoms such as anxiety, depression, and fear are common across the treatment trajectory. Nurses use therapeutic communication to identify early emotional distress. Collaboration with psychologists and social workers ensures timely intervention. Activities like art therapy, journaling, and play support expression and coping. Nurses foster resilience by reinforcing positive coping behaviors and family cohesion. Education includes normalizing emotional fluctuations and encouraging open dialogue. Compassionate listening validates feelings and reduces isolation. Addressing mental health is essential to comprehensive symptom management.

Cognitive and Learning Changes

Treatment-related neurocognitive effects may include attention deficits and slower information processing. Nurses collaborate with educators to provide academic accommodations and individualized education plans. Early neuropsychological evaluation helps identify deficits and guide interventions. Cognitive rehabilitation exercises support gradual improvement. Education for parents highlights patience and consistent reinforcement at home. Nurses coordinate communication among teachers, therapists, and families to ensure consistency. Recognition and early intervention mitigate long-term academic challenges. Advocacy for continued learning opportunities supports the child's self-esteem and future potential.

Growth, Development, and Hormonal Balance

Chronic illness and therapy may impede growth and development. Nurses track height, weight, and developmental milestones to identify deviations. Education for families emphasizes balanced nutrition and adherence to hormone therapies when prescribed. Collaboration with endocrinologists ensures appropriate monitoring and replacement regimens. Emotional support for children experiencing delayed growth or puberty fosters self-acceptance. Encouraging participation in normal activities maintains social and emotional growth. Developmental care strategies promote age-appropriate autonomy and adaptation. Addressing growth comprehensively ensures lifelong wellness and confidence.

Supportive Care

Medical Devices and Infusion Safety

Use of central venous catheters, ports, and infusion pumps is integral to therapy. Nurses ensure sterile technique during access and maintenance to prevent infection. Education for caregivers includes flushing protocols, dressing changes, and recognition of complications such as occlusion or leakage. Vigilance for signs of extravasation or dislodgment prevents severe tissue injury. Safety checks before medication delivery uphold reliability. Teaching promotes family confidence in home device management. Proper device care ensures continuity of therapy without interruption.

Blood Product Administration and Colony-Stimulating Factors

Supportive therapy often involves transfusions and administration of hematopoietic growth factors. Nurses verify compatibility, monitor for transfusion reactions, and document responses precisely. Education includes signs of delayed reactions and follow-up laboratory assessments. Growth factors require awareness of potential side effects such as bone pain or spleen enlargement. Nurses evaluate tolerance and adjust care plans accordingly. Clear communication fosters trust and compliance. These supportive measures sustain hematologic stability during intensive treatment.

Interdisciplinary and Palliative Collaboration

Palliative care integrates symptom relief and emotional support throughout the illness course, not only at the end of life. Nurses collaborate with interdisciplinary teams to address pain, fatigue, and psychological distress. Open dialogue with families ensures alignment of care goals. Nurses help coordinate community resources such as counseling, spiritual care, and respite services. Compassionate presence during decision-making fosters peace and understanding. This holistic approach ensures comfort and dignity for the child and family. Collaborative teamwork transforms suffering into meaningful, supported care.

Complementary and Integrative Modalities

Integrative approaches such as relaxation therapy, music, massage, and acupuncture may alleviate symptoms and enhance well-being. Nurses assess safety and evidence before recommending complementary methods. Families receive guidance on combining these therapies with medical treatment responsibly. Monitoring for adverse reactions ensures protection from harmful interactions. The nurse respects cultural preferences while reinforcing evidence-based practice. Encouraging holistic care improves emotional balance and comfort. Integrative modalities complement traditional medicine, enhancing overall quality of life.

Nutrition, Hydration, and Metabolic Support

Adequate nutrition and hydration remain vital during all phases of treatment. Nurses assess intake, tolerance, and metabolic needs. Dietary modifications address taste changes and nausea. Enteral or parenteral nutrition may be required to meet caloric demands. Education for families focuses on food safety, portion management, and hydration cues. Collaboration with dietitians ensures individualized support. Maintaining metabolic stability promotes recovery and resilience. Sustained attention to nutrition strengthens every aspect of healing.

Family Education and Advocacy

Families are central to supportive care, serving as partners in symptom management. Nurses provide clear explanations of care routines, medication schedules, and emergency responses. Education is delivered through repetition, demonstration, and reassurance. Advocacy ensures that family preferences and concerns shape the plan of care. Encouraging open communication builds mutual respect and collaboration. Nurses empower families to voice questions and participate confidently. Active partnership transforms supportive care into shared healing.

Chapter-5: Pediatric Hematologic and Oncologic Emergencies

Infectious Emergencies

Recognition and Early Intervention

Infection remains one of the most serious and life-threatening complications in pediatric hematology and oncology. Children undergoing chemotherapy or post–stem cell transplant are profoundly immunocompromised, making even minor infections potentially fatal. Nurses monitor temperature trends, neutrophil counts, and early clinical signs such as lethargy or tachycardia. Rapid assessment and immediate notification of the medical team are critical when fever or suspected sepsis arises. Timely initiation of empiric antibiotics prevents septic shock and organ failure. Education for families emphasizes strict hand hygiene and the importance of seeking care at the first sign of fever. The nurse also evaluates environmental factors, ensuring cleanliness in hospital and home settings. Vigilance and swift action remain the cornerstone of infection control in immunosuppressed children.

Sepsis Management and Hemodynamic Support

Sepsis requires prompt fluid resuscitation, antibiotic administration, and hemodynamic stabilization. Nurses assess perfusion, capillary refill, and urine output continuously. Early goal-directed therapy ensures oxygen delivery to vital organs. Monitoring for signs of septic shock such as hypotension or altered mental status allows for immediate escalation of care. The nurse coordinates with critical care teams for vasopressor support if indicated. Laboratory results guide ongoing therapy, including cultures and inflammatory markers. Education for families focuses on understanding the urgency of sepsis symptoms. Compassionate reassurance and clear communication sustain family confidence during this critical phase.

Neutropenic Precautions and Isolation

During periods of profound neutropenia, preventive care becomes paramount. Nurses implement protective isolation, strict hand hygiene, and environmental cleaning. Visitors are screened for illness, and caregivers receive guidance on food safety and personal protective equipment. Central line care and daily assessments for mucosal integrity reduce infection entry points. Education reinforces the importance of avoiding crowds and monitoring for early symptoms. Nurses document adherence to protocols and evaluate effectiveness. These interventions dramatically decrease infection-related morbidity. Maintaining isolation safety preserves patient well-being without compromising emotional support.

Typhlitis and Gastrointestinal Infections

Typhlitis, or neutropenic enterocolitis, presents with abdominal pain, fever, and diarrhea. It is a medical emergency requiring immediate intervention. Nurses assess bowel sounds, distension, and tenderness while monitoring vital signs and laboratory markers. Supportive care includes bowel rest, IV fluids, and broad-spectrum antibiotics. Education for families highlights recognizing early gastrointestinal symptoms. Collaboration with the medical team ensures timely imaging and surgical consultation when necessary. Gentle reassurance reduces fear while emphasizing the seriousness of symptoms. Vigilant nursing observation prevents complications such as perforation or sepsis.

Infection Prevention in the Home Environment

Upon discharge, infection prevention shifts to the home setting. Nurses educate caregivers on maintaining clean surroundings, proper food handling, and avoiding exposure to infectious contacts. Safe pet practices and environmental monitoring are reinforced. The nurse provides guidelines on temperature monitoring and when to contact healthcare providers. Ongoing communication through follow-up calls supports adherence. Families are encouraged to keep emergency contact numbers accessible. Consistent education empowers families to sustain infection control outside the hospital. Home safety becomes a shared responsibility that protects the child's recovery.

Fungal and Opportunistic Infections

Immunosuppression increases vulnerability to fungal and opportunistic pathogens. Nurses monitor for persistent fever, respiratory distress, or new lesions suggestive of fungal involvement. Early identification and prompt antifungal therapy improve survival. Education covers medication adherence, potential side effects, and the importance of consistent follow-up. Collaboration with infectious disease specialists ensures individualized management. Environmental precautions, such as avoiding construction areas and mold exposure, are emphasized. Supportive care balances antimicrobial efficacy with minimizing toxicity. Continuous surveillance ensures protection against silent, invasive infections.

Metabolic Emergencies

Tumor Lysis Syndrome

Tumor lysis syndrome results from rapid tumor cell breakdown releasing potassium, phosphate, and uric acid into circulation. Nurses monitor for signs of renal failure, arrhythmias, and electrolyte imbalances. Preventive care includes aggressive hydration and administration of allopurinol or rasburicase. Continuous cardiac monitoring detects early arrhythmias. Education for families highlights the importance of hydration and laboratory monitoring during induction therapy. The nurse collaborates with laboratory staff to interpret critical results promptly. Intervention with IV fluids, diuretics, and electrolyte management prevents complications. Early recognition ensures safety during high-risk treatment initiation.

Syndrome of Inappropriate Antidiuretic Hormone (SIADH)

SIADH presents with hyponatremia, decreased urine output, and neurological symptoms. Nurses monitor fluid balance, serum sodium, and neurological status. Management includes fluid restriction and medication adjustment. Education for families focuses on recognizing confusion, headache, or seizures. Collaboration with the medical team ensures timely intervention to prevent cerebral edema. The nurse reinforces adherence to fluid limits and monitors tolerance. Empathetic communication helps families understand the delicate balance of fluid management. Vigilance prevents severe neurological complications and supports recovery.

Hypercalcemia of Malignancy

Hypercalcemia results from bone metastasis or paraneoplastic syndromes. Nurses assess for fatigue, dehydration, constipation, and confusion. Interventions include IV hydration, diuretics, and bisphosphonate therapy. Monitoring calcium levels and renal function ensures response to treatment. Education for families addresses maintaining fluid intake and recognizing early symptoms. Emotional reassurance helps manage anxiety associated with altered mental status. Collaboration with dietitians and physicians optimizes supportive care. Timely management prevents cardiac and renal complications.

Diabetes Insipidus and Electrolyte Imbalance

Diabetes insipidus may occur after cranial irradiation or tumor involvement of the hypothalamus. Nurses monitor urine output, specific gravity, and hydration status. Administration of desmopressin and fluid replacement stabilizes balance. Families learn to recognize excessive thirst or urination as warning signs. The nurse provides education on medication adherence and emergency planning. Documentation of trends supports physician decision-making. Maintaining electrolyte stability prevents dehydration crises. Consistent monitoring ensures safety and comfort.

Cytokine Release Syndrome

Cytokine release syndrome may accompany cellular therapies like CAR-T cell treatment. Symptoms include fever, hypotension, and respiratory distress. Nurses monitor vital signs frequently and assess for escalating severity using standardized grading scales. Early intervention with corticosteroids or tocilizumab can prevent progression to organ failure. Families are educated on recognizing symptoms at home post-infusion. Coordination with critical care teams ensures readiness for rapid response. Emotional reassurance alleviates fear during acute reactions. Skilled nursing assessment is vital for survival during this therapy.

Multidisciplinary Response to Metabolic Crises

Metabolic emergencies demand a collaborative response involving physicians, pharmacists, dietitians, and laboratory professionals. Nurses facilitate communication and implement treatment plans promptly. Accurate documentation supports timely evaluation of interventions. Education for caregivers focuses on emergency recognition and quick reporting. Emotional support during crises maintains family stability. Collaboration ensures that no aspect of care is delayed. This coordinated approach reflects the highest standard of pediatric oncology practice.

Vascular Emergencies

Disseminated Intravascular Coagulation (DIC)

DIC involves widespread clotting and bleeding due to uncontrolled activation of coagulation pathways. Nurses monitor for bruising, petechiae, and prolonged bleeding times. Interventions include transfusion of platelets, plasma, or cryoprecipitate. Frequent vital signs and laboratory assessments track disease progression. Education for families highlights early signs of bleeding and need for prompt reporting. Maintaining safety through gentle handling and minimal invasive procedures prevents trauma. Emotional support reduces distress during intensive monitoring. Vigilant nursing care ensures rapid stabilization and improved outcomes.

Thrombosis and Hyperleukocytosis

Thrombosis and hyperleukocytosis increase risk for stroke, pulmonary embolism, and organ infarction. Nurses assess neurological status, oxygenation, and perfusion regularly. Immediate notification of abnormal findings initiates emergency management such as leukapheresis or anticoagulation therapy. Education for families includes recognizing sudden weakness or breathing difficulty. Preventive measures such as adequate hydration and mobility reduce risk. Emotional reassurance helps families remain calm during urgent interventions. Coordination with hematology teams ensures rapid response and safety. Proactive monitoring prevents life-threatening complications.

Hemorrhage and Splenic Sequestration

Severe bleeding and splenic sequestration may occur in conditions like sickle cell disease or leukemia. Nurses assess for pallor, abdominal distension, and hypotension. Prompt intervention includes transfusion support and fluid resuscitation. Family education focuses on recognizing abdominal pain or sudden weakness. Nurses ensure transfusion safety and monitor response. Collaboration with medical teams facilitates rapid stabilization. Emotional support reassures families facing recurrent crises. Preventive education on early recognition significantly improves outcomes.

Sinusoidal Obstructive Syndrome

This condition results from hepatic injury due to chemotherapy or stem cell transplantation. Nurses monitor for jaundice, weight gain, and hepatomegaly. Early intervention includes fluid restriction, diuretics, and pain management. Families receive education on monitoring abdominal girth and reporting discomfort. Collaboration with hepatologists and transplant specialists ensures coordinated care. Documentation of fluid balance supports medical decision-making. Compassionate explanations help families understand the condition’s seriousness. Diligent monitoring preserves organ function and patient comfort.

Stroke and Neurological Events

Stroke presents with weakness, facial droop, or altered speech. Nurses initiate emergency protocols for rapid imaging and supportive management. Prevention includes hydration, transfusions, and monitoring hemoglobin levels in at-risk patients. Education for families emphasizes early recognition and the importance of immediate care. Post-stroke rehabilitation involves collaboration with physical and occupational therapists. Emotional support helps families adjust to neurological deficits. Nurses advocate for long-term follow-up and secondary prevention strategies. Consistent assessment reduces recurrence risk and improves recovery.

Joint Bleeds and Musculoskeletal Emergencies

Joint bleeds, especially in hemophilia, cause pain, swelling, and limited mobility. Nurses apply immobilization and administer clotting factors promptly. Pain management includes rest, cold compresses, and gentle positioning. Education for caregivers focuses on preventing re-injury and maintaining safe play activities. Collaboration with physiotherapists supports rehabilitation once bleeding resolves. Emotional reassurance promotes confidence in activity resumption. Preventive education reduces chronic joint damage and enhances quality of life.

Neurological and Cardiopulmonary Emergencies

Increased Intracranial Pressure

Increased intracranial pressure may result from tumor growth, hemorrhage, or infection. Nurses monitor neurological status, pupil reaction, and vital signs for early changes. Elevating the head of the bed and minimizing stimuli reduce pressure. Collaboration with physicians ensures rapid administration of corticosteroids or diuretics. Families receive clear explanations of symptoms and treatments. Emotional support helps manage fear during critical care interventions. Ongoing observation ensures timely intervention and preservation of neurological function.

Seizure Management

Seizures require immediate safety measures including airway protection and injury prevention. Nurses administer antiepileptic medications and monitor for side effects. Education for families covers medication adherence and seizure first aid. Identifying triggers helps reduce recurrence. Emotional reassurance and postictal care promote recovery. Documentation includes duration and characteristics to guide medical decisions. Comprehensive management ensures both safety and emotional stability.

Respiratory Distress and Pleural Effusion

Respiratory distress can occur due to mediastinal masses or pleural effusion. Nurses assess breathing patterns, oxygen saturation, and anxiety levels. Immediate interventions include positioning, oxygen administration, and notification of the medical team. Education for families emphasizes recognizing signs of worsening distress. Collaboration with respiratory therapists ensures proper airway management. Emotional support during acute episodes reduces fear. Continuous monitoring provides early warning of deterioration.

Acute Chest Syndrome

Common in sickle cell disease, acute chest syndrome presents with fever, chest pain, and hypoxia. Nurses prioritize oxygen therapy, antibiotic administration, and incentive spirometry. Pain control facilitates breathing and recovery. Education reinforces adherence to treatment and hydration. Collaboration with the medical team ensures coordinated care. Emotional reassurance supports families through recurrent crises. Vigilance reduces morbidity and prevents recurrence.

Cardiac Arrhythmias and Toxicity

Chemotherapy agents may cause arrhythmias and cardiomyopathy. Nurses monitor cardiac rhythm, blood pressure, and drug compatibility. Education for families includes recognizing palpitations or dizziness. Collaboration with cardiologists ensures accurate assessment and timely intervention. Documentation of cumulative drug doses aids in risk monitoring. Emotional support alleviates fear during cardiac evaluations. Regular surveillance maintains cardiovascular safety throughout therapy.

Anaphylaxis and Hypersensitivity Reactions

Anaphylaxis can develop suddenly during drug infusion. Nurses must recognize early signs such as rash, wheezing, or hypotension. Emergency response includes stopping the infusion, administering epinephrine, and providing airway support. Families are educated about allergy identification and use of emergency kits. Preparation and readiness ensure prompt action. Continuous monitoring after stabilization detects biphasic reactions. Emotional reassurance and follow-up teaching reinforce confidence. Rapid response and prevention save lives during hypersensitivity events.

Chapter-6: Psychosocial Dimensions of Care

Social Relationships and Family Dynamics

Impact of Illness on Family Systems

A pediatric cancer diagnosis disrupts every aspect of family life, introducing fear, uncertainty, and financial strain. Parents may struggle to balance caregiving responsibilities with work obligations, while siblings often experience feelings of neglect or guilt. Nurses assess family structure, communication styles, and coping capacity to tailor interventions appropriately. Family meetings create opportunities for open dialogue and collaborative problem-solving. Encouraging parents to share responsibilities and maintain routines fosters stability and resilience. Nurses promote inclusion of siblings in discussions to reduce anxiety and misunderstanding. Education focuses on realistic expectations and available community resources. Addressing family stress proactively helps preserve emotional equilibrium. The nurse's presence as a consistent, empathetic professional provides reassurance during the turbulence of treatment.

Support for Parents and Caregivers

Parents often experience intense emotional exhaustion and decision-making fatigue. Nurses offer emotional support, education, and referrals to counseling or support groups. Caregivers benefit from structured teaching on symptom management, medication administration, and self-care strategies. Encouraging rest, nutrition, and peer connection strengthens caregiver endurance. Nurses help identify burnout early by monitoring for irritability, withdrawal, or hopelessness. Providing flexible education formats—written, verbal, or digital—accommodates varying levels of stress and comprehension. Empowering caregivers enhances their confidence and engagement. Compassionate guidance helps them sustain nurturing relationships while managing medical demands.

Sibling and Peer Relationships

Siblings of ill children may feel isolated, frightened, or jealous due to attention shifts within the family. Nurses assess sibling understanding and emotional well-being, offering age-appropriate education about the illness. Encouraging sibling visits when safe and maintaining open communication reduces confusion and fear. Peer relationships for the patient are equally vital; maintaining school contact or digital communication prevents social isolation. Nurses collaborate with child life specialists to facilitate safe play and peer interaction. Providing guidance to parents on including siblings in care decisions fosters family unity. Supporting sibling resilience contributes to holistic family recovery.

Reintegration into Family, School, and Community Life

Returning home or to school after intensive treatment requires coordinated planning. Nurses collaborate with educators to ensure accommodations such as reduced workloads or modified schedules. Family education covers infection precautions, fatigue management, and psychosocial support during reintegration. The nurse encourages gradual reintroduction to activities that promote normalcy and confidence. Emotional preparation for social re-entry helps children address changes in appearance or ability. Advocacy ensures that schools and communities foster understanding and inclusion. Continuous communication between home and hospital teams ensures consistent support. Reintegration symbolizes recovery not only from disease but also from emotional isolation.

Cultural and Family Values in Care

Cultural beliefs strongly influence family perceptions of illness, decision-making, and coping strategies. Nurses conduct culturally sensitive assessments that respect traditions, language preferences, and faith practices. Incorporating spiritual support and interpreters ensures inclusivity. Family rituals may provide comfort and meaning during hospitalization. Nurses advocate for culturally appropriate accommodations whenever possible, fostering trust. Education materials are tailored to linguistic and literacy needs.

Sensitivity to family values enhances cooperation and adherence to care plans. Recognizing culture as a strength empowers families to participate fully in healing.

Socioeconomic Challenges and Resource Connection

Financial strain from medical bills, transportation, and work absence often compounds family stress. Nurses identify resource needs early and collaborate with social workers to secure assistance programs. Community organizations, grants, and charitable funds can provide relief for nonmedical expenses. Nurses help families navigate insurance complexities and hospital billing systems. Emotional support acknowledges the dignity of families facing hardship. Access to nutrition, housing, and psychological support stabilizes the caregiving environment. Advocacy for equitable resource access reflects the nurse's commitment to holistic care. Addressing socioeconomic needs strengthens the foundation for recovery.

Principles of Growth and Development

Developmentally Sensitive Communication

Understanding the child's developmental stage guides effective communication. Young children benefit from concrete explanations and play-based demonstrations, while adolescents prefer honest, autonomy-respecting dialogue. Nurses use therapeutic play, visual aids, and storytelling to reduce anxiety. Consistent and transparent communication builds trust across age groups. The nurse reassures children by maintaining predictable routines and consistent caregivers. Encouraging questions helps children express fears and gain control. Communication that matches developmental understanding enhances cooperation and comfort during care.

Cognitive and Emotional Milestones

Illness and treatment can delay or alter developmental progress. Nurses monitor cognitive skills, social behavior, and emotional expression throughout therapy. Collaboration with psychologists and educators supports ongoing learning and adjustment. Interventions such as memory games, creative art, or group play encourage continued development. Family education helps parents provide supportive stimulation at home. Early identification of regression or delayed milestones prompts timely therapy referrals. Promoting age-appropriate independence strengthens confidence. Developmental vigilance ensures balanced growth despite medical challenges.

Play and Therapeutic Activities

Play remains a vital tool for expression, coping, and learning. Nurses encourage play therapy tailored to treatment context—using dolls to explain procedures or art to express emotions. Playrooms or bedside activities reduce fear and isolation during hospitalization. Structured play sessions promote normalcy and emotional release. Collaboration with child life specialists enhances therapeutic outcomes. Family participation in play strengthens bonds and reduces stress. Through play, children regain a sense of control and continuity in daily life.

Adolescent Identity and Autonomy

Adolescents face unique psychosocial stressors as they navigate independence, peer relationships, and body image. Nurses respect privacy, involve teens in decision-making, and support self-advocacy. Honest communication about fertility, sexuality, and long-term effects fosters trust. Encouraging social connections through support groups or online communities reduces isolation. Nurses monitor for risk behaviors that may stem from emotional distress. Supporting autonomy within safe boundaries promotes resilience. Recognizing adolescence as a developmental turning point ensures care that respects both individuality and dependence.

School and Education Continuity

Maintaining educational continuity supports cognitive and emotional well-being. Nurses coordinate with school systems to arrange home or hospital instruction. Liaising between teachers, counselors, and healthcare providers ensures accommodations for fatigue and absences. Education plans should reflect medical limitations while promoting achievable goals. Emotional preparation for school reintegration includes addressing peer curiosity and self-image. Advocacy for educational equality empowers long-term academic success. Collaboration between family, school, and healthcare teams preserves a child's sense of purpose and identity.

Transition Between Developmental Phases

Each stage of growth requires adaptation in nursing care and family support. Nurses anticipate changing needs as children mature, from dependency in early childhood to autonomy in adolescence. Education for parents includes understanding these transitions and adjusting expectations. Interventions evolve to promote independence, responsibility, and resilience. Encouraging life skills such as decision-making and communication prepares youth for adulthood. Emotional guidance supports both child and family through evolving roles. Developmentally aligned care nurtures confidence and lifelong adaptability.

Grief and Bereavement

Understanding Pediatric Grief

Children experience grief differently based on age, development, and personal experience. Nurses observe behavioral cues such as withdrawal, aggression, or regression as expressions of loss. Clear, honest explanations about death support comprehension and reduce fear. Encouraging emotional expression through art or play allows children to process feelings safely. Nurses create an atmosphere where grief is normalized and supported. Sensitivity to cultural and spiritual interpretations of death enhances comfort. Recognizing individual grief patterns allows for tailored interventions. Compassionate guidance transforms grief into healing.

Parental Bereavement and Emotional Recovery

Parents grieving a child's illness or death experience profound emotional devastation. Nurses provide nonjudgmental presence, active listening, and referrals to bereavement counseling. Encouraging memory-making activities such as keepsakes or letters supports meaning-making. Nurses respect diverse grieving processes and avoid imposing timelines for recovery. Connecting families with peer support groups reduces isolation. Follow-up communication after loss demonstrates continued care. Sensitivity and compassion ensure that families feel valued beyond the patient's life. Grief support remains an enduring nursing responsibility.

Sibling Grief and Adjustment

Siblings often feel confused or abandoned after a sibling's death. Nurses facilitate open discussions using age-appropriate language to clarify misconceptions. Encouraging participation in memorial rituals fosters inclusion and closure. Collaboration with child psychologists and school counselors ensures sustained support. Nurses help parents balance their grief while nurturing surviving children. Providing resources such as sibling support camps promotes healing. Recognizing sibling grief preserves family unity and strengthens long-term adjustment. Each child's grief deserves individual acknowledgment and care.

Staff Support and Compassion Fatigue Prevention

Caring for terminally ill children deeply affects healthcare providers. Nurses may experience secondary trauma or moral distress. Institutions should provide debriefing sessions and access to counseling for staff. Peer support and reflective practice help manage emotional exhaustion. Recognizing limits and seeking support demonstrates professionalism, not weakness. Encouraging work-life balance preserves empathy and effectiveness. Nurturing staff well-being ensures sustained compassionate care for patients and families. Self-care among nurses reinforces the integrity of holistic care.

Spiritual and Cultural Perspectives on Loss

Cultural and spiritual beliefs shape family responses to death and mourning. Nurses respect rituals, prayer practices, and beliefs about the afterlife. Collaboration with chaplains or cultural liaisons ensures inclusive support. Families find comfort in preserving traditions during hospitalization or memorial services. Nurses adapt care practices to honor these preferences respectfully. Encouraging open discussion of faith can provide solace. Sensitivity to belief systems fosters trust and healing. Embracing diversity enhances the human connection at life's most vulnerable moments.

Long-Term Bereavement Follow-Up

Nursing care extends beyond the immediate loss through follow-up calls, letters, or grief counseling referrals. Families appreciate continued recognition of their loved one's memory. Nurses provide resources for ongoing therapy or support groups. Monitoring family adjustment allows early intervention if prolonged grief impairs function. Encouraging self-compassion and community involvement facilitates recovery. Continued contact affirms that care does not end with death. Sustained bereavement support exemplifies the enduring compassion central to pediatric oncology nursing.

Chapter-7: Practice Question

Question (1-100)

Q1. A nurse is planning discharge teaching for a child newly diagnosed with acute lymphoblastic leukemia (ALL). Which strategy best supports the transition from hospital to home care?

A. Provide a list of medications only
B. Schedule a single follow-up appointment
C. Arrange multidisciplinary coordination and family education
D. Give written discharge instructions only

Q2. A nurse caring for a child with sickle cell disease prepares a care plan for home management. Which teaching point is most essential for preventing vaso-occlusive crises?

A. Encourage fluid restriction
B. Promote adequate hydration and rest
C. Limit physical activity entirely
D. Increase protein intake only

Q3. During care transition, a nurse identifies that a patient's home lacks resources for safe chemotherapy administration. What is the most appropriate nursing action?

A. Proceed with discharge and inform the next shift
B. Delay discharge and involve case management
C. Teach parents to manage without additional help
D. Contact pharmacy to adjust dosage

Q4. A child recently completed therapy for Hodgkin lymphoma. Which survivorship plan component is most important for long-term health?

A. Routine imaging every month
B. Limiting physical activity permanently
C. Avoidance of all vaccinations
D. Documentation of treatment summary and late effects monitoring

Q5. When transitioning an adolescent with leukemia from pediatric to adult care, what is the nurse's priority action?

A. Schedule appointments for the parents
B. Discuss self-management and healthcare navigation skills
C. Transfer medical records only
D. Delay transition until adulthood

Q6. A pediatric oncology nurse collaborates with school personnel for a child returning after stem cell transplant. What is the most critical educational point for teachers?

A. Encourage class participation despite fatigue
B. Delay all peer interaction indefinitely
C. Avoid providing academic materials
D. Prevent infection exposure through precautions

Q7. A nurse evaluates a family's ability to manage complex home infusions for a child with hemophilia. Which assessment finding requires additional intervention?

A. Parent demonstrates correct sterile technique
B. Parent expresses fear of causing harm during infusion
C. Supplies are organized and labeled
D. Family maintains emergency contact numbers

Q8. Which strategy best supports health promotion for a child in remission from acute myeloid leukemia (AML)?

A. Annual survivorship visits and vaccination review
B. Avoidance of all school activities
C. Restriction of diet permanently
D. Frequent invasive testing

Q9. During end-of-life care, a nurse coordinates interdisciplinary meetings for a child with relapsed leukemia. What is the primary goal of this collaboration?

A. To decide on curative treatment only
B. To align goals of care and symptom management
C. To reduce family involvement in decisions
D. To focus exclusively on medical interventions

Q10. A nurse supports a family during the transition to hospice care for their child with refractory neuroblastoma. Which nursing action demonstrates best practice?

A. Emphasize discontinuation of all medications
B. Avoid discussing prognosis
C. Encourage ongoing symptom management and emotional support
D. Focus only on hospital-based comfort care

Q11. A nurse is collaborating with a community health nurse to coordinate care for a child discharged after induction therapy for

leukemia. What is the most appropriate priority to address?

A. Scheduling recreational therapy first

B. Establishing infection prevention and monitoring plans

C. Arranging only financial counseling

D. Reducing communication with outpatient staff

Q12. A nurse caring for a child newly diagnosed with thalassemia discusses long-term management with the parents. Which teaching topic is most important at diagnosis?

A. Importance of routine transfusion and iron chelation schedules

B. Avoidance of physical activity

C. Minimizing social contact permanently

D. Reducing follow-up appointments

Q13. A school nurse contacts the oncology team about a child who has completed chemotherapy six months earlier. What is the best guidance regarding immunizations?

A. Administer double vaccine doses

B. Restart all live vaccines immediately

C. Avoid all vaccines for five years

D. Resume routine vaccines after immune recovery is verified

Q14. When planning discharge for a child receiving palliative radiation, which nursing intervention best ensures continuity of symptom control?

A. Provide medication schedule and contact numbers for home support

B. Rely solely on verbal instructions

C. Discontinue all analgesics

D. Schedule follow-up only if pain worsens

Q15. A nurse assists in developing a survivorship plan for a teenager post-osteosarcoma treatment. Which element must be included?

A. Schedule for cardiac and renal monitoring

B. Daily imaging for relapse detection

C. Restriction from future exercise

D. Elimination of all future health screenings

Q16. Parents of a child completing treatment for Wilms' tumor express fear about cancer returning. What is the nurse's best response?

A. Encourage avoiding medical discussions at home

B. Dismiss their anxiety and change the topic

C. Discuss scheduled surveillance visits and normal emotional reactions

D. Provide only written materials without conversation

Q17. A nurse is coordinating outpatient follow-up for a child with a new central venous catheter. Which educational focus is most essential for caregivers?

A. Hand hygiene and line-flushing technique

B. Recognizing only medication names

C. Avoiding line use altogether

D. Removing the dressing weekly

Q18. A nurse caring for a child with hemophilia preparing for home therapy notices the family has difficulty organizing supplies. What is the best nursing intervention?

A. Create a written checklist and storage plan

B. Allow the family to develop their own routine later

C. Store supplies randomly for convenience

D. Cancel discharge until supplies are replaced

Q19. A nurse participates in an interdisciplinary meeting for a child with relapsed leukemia receiving palliative chemotherapy. What should the nurse advocate for during planning?

A. Avoiding psychosocial services

B. Discontinuation of all communication with family

C. Prioritizing curative intent only

D. Integration of symptom control with family goals

Q20. A pediatric oncology nurse reviews a patient's discharge medications and notes an oral chemotherapy agent. Which step ensures safety before release?

A. Verify dosing and educate caregivers on protective handling

B. Provide medication without explanation

C. Instruct family to adjust doses if nausea occurs

D. Delegate teaching to non-clinical staff

Q21. A child with leukemia is being discharged to continue oral mercaptopurine at home. Which instruction should the nurse include to prevent dosing errors?

A. Crush tablets to make them easier to swallow

B. Measure liquid doses carefully using a calibrated syringe

C. Store medication with household supplies
D. Stop medication if mild nausea occurs

Q22. During discharge planning, a nurse notes that parents struggle with organizing follow-up appointments for their child with sickle cell anemia. Which strategy best supports adherence?
A. Create a written calendar of appointments and contact numbers
B. Encourage the family to call when they remember
C. Schedule appointments without notifying parents
D. Provide verbal reminders only

Q23. An adolescent with hemophilia is transitioning from parental to self-care management. What is the most appropriate nursing goal?
A. Teach infusion technique and emergency response readiness
B. Assign all care decisions to parents
C. Restrict patient involvement in care
D. Delay transition until adulthood

Q24. A nurse plans a survivorship visit for a child treated for acute lymphoblastic leukemia (ALL). Which assessment is most important at this stage?
A. Avoid discussing long-term effects
B. Focus only on acute infection symptoms
C. Evaluate growth, endocrine status, and cognitive function
D. Limit assessments to vital signs

Q25. When preparing a family for home management after hematopoietic stem cell transplantation, what education should be prioritized?
A. Infection prevention and environmental control measures
B. Routine use of public transportation
C. Unrestricted social contact
D. Avoidance of all medications

Q26. A nurse caring for a family whose child has completed chemotherapy observes signs of parental exhaustion. What is the best intervention?
A. Offer referral to psychosocial support and respite care
B. Increase medication teaching sessions
C. Encourage the parents to ignore fatigue
D. Provide only written discharge instructions

Q27. A nurse meets with a multidisciplinary team to discuss a child returning home after hospitalization for neutropenic fever. What should the nurse emphasize?
A. Restricting the child to bed rest indefinitely
B. Resuming large social gatherings immediately
C. Avoiding all contact with school staff
D. Consistent handwashing and environmental hygiene at home

Q28. A child with sickle cell disease will travel to a higher altitude region. Which anticipatory guidance should the nurse provide?
A. Maintain hydration and avoid extreme temperatures
B. Reduce fluid intake to prevent nocturia
C. Stop all medications during travel
D. Avoid seeking medical help if pain occurs

Q29. A nurse evaluates understanding of survivorship care among parents of a child cured of lymphoma. Which statement indicates correct understanding?
A. "We will continue regular follow-ups to monitor for late effects."
B. "We don't need to see the doctor again now that treatment is over."
C. "Screenings are unnecessary since the cancer is cured."
D. "We'll only call if new symptoms appear."

Q30. A nurse supporting a family at end-of-life for their child with refractory leukemia should prioritize which action?
A. Emphasize medical decisions only
B. Facilitate open discussion of care preferences and comfort needs
C. Discourage family presence during procedures
D. Avoid emotional conversations

Q31. A nurse teaching about late effects after cranial radiation includes which important concept?
A. Regular neurocognitive and endocrine evaluation
B. No follow-up needed after one year
C. Avoid discussing academic performance
D. Discontinue growth assessments

Q32. A newly diagnosed pediatric oncology patient's family expresses confusion about care

coordination between inpatient and outpatient settings. What should the nurse do?
A. Introduce the case manager and provide a contact list
B. Advise the family to figure out scheduling independently
C. Provide only verbal directions
D. Delay education until discharge
Q33. A child with hemophilia has frequent hospital admissions for joint bleeding. Which health promotion intervention may reduce future episodes?
A. Avoid preventive treatments
B. Limit all physical activity
C. Encourage consistent prophylactic factor replacement therapy
D. Administer factor only after bleeds occur
Q34. A nurse preparing discharge teaching for a child with a mediport focuses on which key point?
A. Maintain site cleanliness and monitor for infection signs
B. Keep dressing off for comfort
C. Flush only if the port is painful
D. Ignore redness unless severe
Q35. A nurse facilitating the transition from oncology to primary care for a long-term survivor should prioritize sharing which document?
A. School attendance records
B. Billing history
C. Daily medication logs only
D. Comprehensive treatment summary and surveillance recommendations
Q36. A nurse caring for a child with terminal neuroblastoma notices the sibling withdrawing from activities. What is the most supportive nursing action?
A. Encourage open discussion and referral to child-life or counseling services
B. Focus attention only on the ill child
C. Discourage sibling questions
D. Avoid involving the sibling in care
Q37. A child newly diagnosed with acute lymphoblastic leukemia presents with fatigue and pallor. Which laboratory finding most likely supports this diagnosis?
A. Elevated platelet count
B. Decreased hemoglobin and hematocrit
C. Increased reticulocyte count
D. Elevated hematocrit
Q38. The nurse reviews the pathophysiology of sickle cell disease. The clinical manifestations result primarily from which mechanism?
A. Platelet aggregation in small vessels
B. Polymerization of abnormal hemoglobin under low oxygen conditions
C. Autoimmune destruction of red blood cells
D. Deficiency of red cell membrane proteins
Q39. During informed-consent teaching for a Phase II pediatric clinical trial, the nurse emphasizes that this phase primarily evaluates what aspect of the new therapy?
A. Drug absorption and metabolism
B. Long-term population safety
C. Therapeutic effectiveness and short-term side effects
D. Comparison with standard therapy in large populations
Q40. The nurse recognizes that Fanconi anemia is characterized by which underlying defect?
A. Abnormal platelet aggregation
B. Chromosomal breakage leading to bone-marrow failure
C. Deficiency of vitamin B12 absorption
D. Decreased synthesis of globin chains
Q41. A nurse teaches parents about laboratory monitoring for a child receiving methotrexate. Which parameter requires the most vigilant follow-up?
A. Platelet count
B. Serum calcium
C. Blood glucose
D. Sodium level
Q42. When reviewing ethical considerations in pediatric oncology research, which principle is upheld by ensuring parents and older children understand participation is voluntary?
A. Fidelity
B. Justice
C. Autonomy
D. Beneficence
Q43. A preschooler with thalassemia major receives frequent transfusions. Which long-term complication is the nurse most concerned about?

A. Hyperkalemia
B. Iron overload
C. Hypocalcemia
D. Neutropenia

Q44. A pediatric oncology nurse encounters conflicting instructions from two physicians regarding chemotherapy dosing. The nurse's best professional action is to:
A. Follow the senior physician's order
B. Delay administration and clarify the discrepancy
C. Choose the smaller dose for safety
D. Ask another nurse to verify and proceed

Q45. Genetic counseling for a family with a child who has retinoblastoma should emphasize what key information?
A. The disorder is exclusively acquired from environmental exposure
B. Siblings have no risk for disease
C. A germline mutation may predispose to bilateral tumors
D. The condition is caused by an infectious agent

Q46. A nurse preparing a teaching session on professional scope of practice should include which statement?
A. It defines the nurse's responsibilities and permissible actions based on licensure and standards
B. It is determined solely by the employing institution
C. It changes with each patient assignment
D. It is optional guidance for advanced nurses

Q47. A nurse is preparing a family for bone-marrow aspiration. Which nursing action best supports atraumatic care?
A. Explaining the procedure only to the parents
B. Allowing the child to choose a coping strategy such as deep breathing
C. Using restraint to prevent movement
D. Avoiding discussion to reduce anxiety

Q48. A nurse notes a child receiving chemotherapy develops petechiae and gum bleeding. Which laboratory value would correlate with these findings?
A. Platelets 15,000/mm^3
B. Hemoglobin 11 g/dL
C. WBC 6,000/mm^3
D. Reticulocytes 2%

Q49. When teaching a new oncology nurse about regulatory standards, which organization is primarily responsible for credentialing the CPHON® certification?
A. American Nurses Association
B. Oncology Nursing Certification Corporation
C. National Cancer Institute
D. American Academy of Pediatrics

Q50. A nurse discusses prognosis with the parents of a child with medulloblastoma. Which statement accurately describes this discussion?
A. It should be avoided until treatment is complete
B. It must balance honesty with sensitivity to emotional readiness
C. It should focus only on statistical outcomes
D. It should be delegated to social work staff

Q51. A child with sickle cell anemia presents with severe pain and swelling in the joints. Which intervention should the nurse prioritize?
A. Administering oxygen therapy
B. Providing intravenous fluids for hydration
C. Applying cold compresses to the joints
D. Giving analgesics for pain management

Q52. A child with leukemia is scheduled for chemotherapy with cyclophosphamide. The nurse explains that a major side effect of this drug is:
A. Cardiotoxicity
B. Renal toxicity
C. Hemorrhagic cystitis
D. Bone marrow suppression

Q53. A nurse is educating a family on the management of a child with hemophilia. Which instruction is most important?
A. Limit physical activity to prevent injury
B. Avoid all vaccinations to reduce risk of bleeding
C. Administer factor replacement therapy as prescribed
D. Encourage high-impact sports for muscle strengthening

Q54. A child receiving chemotherapy develops mouth sores. Which intervention should the nurse recommend to reduce discomfort?
A. Using alcohol-based mouthwash
B. Drinking acidic beverages
C. Encouraging soft, bland foods

D. Administering high doses of vitamin C

Q55. A child receiving methotrexate for cancer treatment is at risk for which potential side effect?

A. Nephrotoxicity
B. Hypoglycemia
C. Hyperkalemia
D. Osteoporosis

Q56. A nurse is reviewing a child's bone marrow biopsy results, which indicate dysplastic changes in erythroid cells. The most likely diagnosis is:

A. Aplastic anemia
B. Sickle cell anemia
C. Myelodysplastic syndrome
D. Iron-deficiency anemia

Q57. A child with leukemia is about to undergo stem cell transplantation. Which is the most critical pre-transplantation care consideration?

A. Assessing pain levels
B. Ensuring emotional support
C. Providing prophylactic antibiotics
D. Reducing environmental stimuli

Q58. A nurse prepares to administer blood products to a child with acute leukemia. Which pre-transfusion action is most important?

A. Administering pain medications
B. Checking the blood type and cross-match
C. Performing a physical exam
D. Educating the family about the procedure

Q59. A nurse is reviewing a child's medication list for a leukemia regimen. The child is prescribed prednisone. What is a common side effect of long-term steroid use in pediatric oncology?

A. Weight loss and anorexia
B. Immunosuppression and infection risk
C. Gastrointestinal bleeding
D. Hypertension and hyperglycemia

Q60. A nurse explains the role of genetic testing for a child diagnosed with retinoblastoma. Which is the most important consideration when interpreting the results of genetic counseling?

A. Risk of hearing loss
B. Risk of secondary cancers in family members
C. Risk of inherited chromosomal abnormalities
D. Risk of environmental causes

Q61. A child receiving chemotherapy is experiencing nausea and vomiting. Which intervention should the nurse prioritize?

A. Administering antiemetic medications as prescribed
B. Reducing fluid intake to avoid bloating
C. Providing high-fat snacks to improve appetite
D. Encouraging the child to avoid eating altogether

Q62. The nurse is reviewing a child's chemotherapy regimen and notices the child is prescribed methotrexate. What is an important nursing consideration with this drug?

A. Monitor for signs of oral ulcers and mucositis
B. Encourage high-sodium foods to prevent fluid retention
C. Educate the child on avoiding vitamin D supplements
D. Ensure the child avoids all vaccines during treatment

Q63. A child with a history of Wilms tumor is in remission and scheduled for routine follow-up. What is a major long-term concern for survivors of this cancer?

A. Growth hormone deficiencies
B. Secondary malignancies due to radiation therapy
C. Allergies to chemotherapy agents
D. Gastrointestinal disorders from abdominal surgery

Q64. A nurse is teaching a family about the side effects of radiation therapy for their child's medulloblastoma. Which of the following should the nurse emphasize?

A. Radiation will have no long-term effects if the child is under 10 years old
B. Cognitive changes may occur due to effects on brain tissue
C. Hair loss is permanent and will not regrow
D. Radiation primarily affects the gastrointestinal system

Q65. A nurse is reviewing the medication list for a child with acute leukemia. The child is prescribed leucovorin. What is the purpose of leucovorin in chemotherapy?

A. To prevent bone marrow suppression
B. To rescue normal cells from the toxic effects of methotrexate

C. To treat chemotherapy-induced nausea and vomiting
D. To enhance the effects of methotrexate on tumor cells

Q66. A child with a history of Hodgkin lymphoma is receiving radiation therapy. What is the primary concern for this patient in the long term?
A. Thyroid dysfunction due to radiation exposure
B. Liver toxicity
C. Hearing loss
D. Renal impairment

Q67. A child with a hematologic malignancy is receiving chemotherapy. Which of the following is the most common long-term effect of chemotherapy in children?
A. Chronic lung disease
B. Secondary cancers
C. Renal failure
D. Cardiac arrhythmias

Q68. A nurse is assessing a child with leukemia receiving chemotherapy. Which lab result would be most concerning?
A. Hemoglobin 10 g/dL
B. White blood cell count 1,500/mm^3
C. Platelet count 100,000/mm^3
D. Serum creatinine 1.0 mg/dL

Q69. A nurse is educating the parents of a child with non-Hodgkin lymphoma on potential side effects of chemotherapy. What should the nurse emphasize?
A. Risk of high blood pressure from steroids
B. Increased risk of infections due to immunosuppression
C. Likely weight gain due to high-calorie treatments
D. Risk of excessive bleeding from low platelet counts

Q70. A child with leukemia is receiving chemotherapy that includes daunorubicin. Which organ toxicity is a primary concern with this drug?
A. Heart
B. Liver
C. Kidneys
D. Lungs

Q71. A child with Hodgkin lymphoma is undergoing radiation therapy. What is the nurse's primary concern during treatment?
A. Risk of bone marrow suppression
B. Development of second cancers in the future
C. Acute allergic reaction to radiation
D. Altered mental status during treatment

Q72. A child with leukemia receiving chemotherapy is found to have neutropenia. What is the nurse's most important intervention?
A. Administer a blood transfusion
B. Increase fluid intake to 2000 mL per day
C. Implement strict hand hygiene and infection precautions
D. Encourage high-fiber foods to promote bowel regularity

Q73. A child receiving chemotherapy is experiencing nausea and vomiting. Which antiemetic should the nurse administer based on the physician's order?
A. Diphenhydramine
B. Ondansetron
C. Lorazepam
D. Methylprednisolone

Q74. The nurse is caring for a child with hemophilia who is experiencing a joint bleed. What is the most important intervention?
A. Apply heat to the affected area
B. Elevate the affected joint and apply ice
C. Perform range-of-motion exercises immediately
D. Restrict the child's physical activity for one week

Q75. A nurse is teaching a family about oral care for a child undergoing chemotherapy. What should be included in the teaching?
A. Use of alcohol-based mouthwash to kill bacteria
B. Avoidance of all liquids during chemotherapy
C. Gentle brushing with a soft toothbrush and use of non-alcoholic mouthwash
D. Regular dental cleanings every two weeks

Q76. A child with sickle cell disease is admitted with pain, fever, and swelling of the joints. The nurse suspects a vaso-occlusive crisis. What is the priority action?
A. Administer blood transfusion

B. Provide pain management and hydration
C. Prepare the child for surgery
D. Give high-dose corticosteroids

Q77. A nurse is caring for a child who is about to receive methotrexate for leukemia. What should the nurse monitor closely before starting therapy?

A. Electrolyte levels
B. Liver function tests
C. Blood glucose levels
D. Platelet count

Q78. A child with acute lymphoblastic leukemia (ALL) is receiving intrathecal chemotherapy. Which is the main purpose of this treatment?

A. To kill leukemic cells in the bone marrow
B. To manage pain related to chemotherapy side effects
C. To reduce the child's overall risk of infection
D. To prevent leukemic cells from infiltrating the central nervous system

Q79. A nurse is reviewing a child's medication list and notices that the child has been prescribed vincristine. What is the most common side effect of this drug?

A. Cardiac arrhythmias
B. Neurotoxicity
C. Hemorrhagic cystitis
D. Pulmonary toxicity

Q80. A nurse is providing discharge teaching for a child with thalassemia. Which instruction should the nurse prioritize?

A. Encouraging high-fat foods to increase weight gain
B. Avoiding iron-rich foods due to the risk of iron overload
C. Restricting fluid intake to prevent heart failure
D. Recommending daily aspirin to reduce blood viscosity

Q81. A nurse is caring for a child receiving a blood transfusion. The nurse notices signs of an allergic reaction. What is the first action the nurse should take?

A. Slow the transfusion rate
B. Stop the transfusion and notify the provider
C. Administer antihistamines as prescribed
D. Monitor vital signs for the next 30 minutes

Q82. A child with a bone marrow disorder is receiving hematopoietic stem cell transplantation. Which is the nurse's priority concern post-transplant?

A. Preventing graft-versus-host disease (GVHD)
B. Ensuring adequate nutrition and hydration
C. Monitoring for signs of graft rejection
D. Supporting the child's emotional well-being

Q83. A nurse is providing discharge instructions to the family of a child who has undergone chemotherapy. Which instruction is most important?

A. Avoid all physical activity for at least one month
B. Keep the child away from crowds and sick individuals
C. Administer over-the-counter medications for any fever
D. Limit oral fluids to avoid overhydration

Q84. A child with leukemia is receiving allopurinol for tumor lysis syndrome. What is the primary purpose of this medication?

A. To reduce hypercalcemia
B. To increase red blood cell production
C. To prevent kidney damage from uric acid crystals
D. To improve bone marrow function

Q85. A nurse is caring for a child with leukemia who is experiencing fatigue. What is the most appropriate action to help manage this symptom?

A. Administer prescribed stimulant medications
B. Encourage short periods of rest throughout the day
C. Increase physical activity to improve stamina
D. Limit fluid intake to reduce the need for rest

Q86. A nurse is caring for a child with leukemia who has developed severe mucositis. What is the best way to manage this condition?

A. Encourage the child to eat hard, crunchy foods to stimulate oral health
B. Provide a bland, soft diet and regular mouth rinses with saline
C. Administer vitamin C to promote healing of the mouth sores
D. Restrict all oral intake to reduce irritation

Q87. A child with sickle cell anemia presents with a pain crisis. What should the nurse prioritize in the management of this condition?

A. Administering oxygen therapy and pain relief

B. Administering blood transfusions
C. Encouraging physical activity to prevent blood stasis
D. Limiting fluid intake to prevent swelling

Q88. A child with leukemia is receiving radiation therapy. What is a common long-term complication of this treatment?
A. Osteoporosis
B. Development of secondary cancers
C. Hearing loss
D. Renal failure

Q89. A child with hemophilia is undergoing a procedure. What is the nurse's first priority before the procedure?
A. Administering pain medication
B. Providing factor replacement therapy
C. Ensuring that the child has fasted for at least 6 hours
D. Applying a pressure dressing to the affected area

Q90. A child with leukemia is receiving chemotherapy and has developed neutropenia. What should the nurse instruct the family to do to prevent infection?
A. Avoid any physical contact with the child
B. Administer antibiotics every day as prescribed
C. Keep the child away from anyone with a cold or infection
D. Encourage the child to participate in group activities

Q91. A child with leukemia is receiving methotrexate therapy. What is a common side effect of this medication that the nurse should monitor for?
A. Hyperkalemia
B. Hepatotoxicity
C. Nephrotoxicity
D. Ototoxicity

Q92. A child with sickle cell disease presents with a painful crisis. What is the first priority in managing this condition?
A. Administering blood transfusions
B. Providing intravenous fluids and pain relief
C. Initiating oxygen therapy
D. Preparing for a splenectomy

Q93. A child with leukemia is receiving intravenous chemotherapy. The nurse notices signs of anaphylaxis during the infusion. What is the nurse's first action?
A. Stop the infusion and administer antihistamines
B. Begin oxygen therapy and prepare for a blood transfusion
C. Increase the infusion rate to flush the drug out of the system
D. Administer epinephrine and stop the infusion

Q94. A nurse is preparing a child with leukemia for a bone marrow biopsy. Which intervention will help minimize the child's anxiety?
A. Encouraging the child to remain silent during the procedure
B. Offering a toy or blanket for comfort during the procedure
C. Using a restraint to prevent movement during the procedure
D. Avoiding any discussion about the procedure to reduce fear

Q95. A child is being treated with vincristine for leukemia. Which adverse effect is the nurse most likely to observe?
A. Constipation and paralytic ileus
B. Renal toxicity and proteinuria
C. Cardiotoxicity and arrhythmias
D. Hearing loss and tinnitus

Q96. A nurse is caring for a child with thalassemia who is receiving regular blood transfusions. What is a long-term complication the nurse should monitor for?
A. Iron overload leading to organ damage
B. Hypocalcemia causing bone fractures
C. Hyperkalemia resulting in cardiac arrhythmias
D. Leukocytosis leading to an increased infection risk

Q97. A nurse is teaching a family about the care of a child with hemophilia. What is the most important instruction to provide?
A. Avoid physical activity to prevent injury
B. Administer factor replacement therapy as prescribed
C. Ensure the child receives regular immunizations
D. Restrict the child’s fluid intake to avoid swelling

Q98. A nurse is assessing a child with leukemia who is receiving high-dose corticosteroid

therapy. What is the most common side effect of this treatment?

A. Osteoporosis and fractures

B. Hyperglycemia and fluid retention

C. Diarrhea and gastrointestinal bleeding

D. Severe allergic reactions and skin rashes

Q99. A child with acute lymphoblastic leukemia (ALL) is undergoing induction chemotherapy. Which lab result should the nurse monitor closely during this phase?

A. Hemoglobin and hematocrit levels

B. Liver function tests

C. White blood cell count and absolute neutrophil count

D. Serum electrolytes

Q100. A nurse is caring for a child receiving chemotherapy with cyclophosphamide. Which side effect should the nurse closely monitor for?

A. Urinary retention

B. Hemorrhagic cystitis

C. Cardiomyopathy

D. Hepatitis

Answer Key and Explanation (1-100)

Q1. Answer: C

Explanation: Transition from hospital to home requires collaboration among healthcare disciplines, including nursing, pharmacy, and social work. Educating the family about medication schedules, infection prevention, and follow-up is vital to continuity. This approach empowers caregivers, reduces complications, and supports safe home management. Coordination ensures each aspect of care is addressed systematically.

Q2. Answer: B

Explanation: Maintaining hydration decreases blood viscosity and helps prevent occlusion of vessels. Adequate rest reduces metabolic demand and tissue hypoxia, lowering crisis risk. Families must understand signs of dehydration and crisis onset. Consistent preventive education supports long-term stability and quality of life.

Q3. Answer: B

Explanation: Safe care transition requires verifying that the home environment can support therapy needs. The nurse must collaborate with case management to arrange resources or home nursing. Discharging without adequate support increases the risk of medication errors or infection. Addressing barriers before discharge ensures patient safety and adherence.

Q4. Answer: D

Explanation: A comprehensive treatment summary allows for tracking potential late effects, secondary malignancies, and fertility issues. It ensures primary care providers understand prior therapies and their implications. Periodic health evaluations and surveillance are coordinated based on this summary. Such documentation is foundational to survivorship care planning.

Q5. Answer: B

Explanation: Transition readiness includes promoting autonomy, medication management, and understanding health history. Early education enables adolescents to engage in their own care confidently. Successful transition depends on communication among pediatric and adult teams. Preparing the patient ensures continuity and adherence to long-term monitoring.

Q6. Answer: D

Explanation: Post-transplant immunosuppression places children at high infection risk. School staff must understand hand hygiene, symptom recognition, and exclusion during outbreaks. Safe reintegration allows psychosocial recovery while maintaining health precautions. Collaboration ensures both educational and medical needs are met.

Q7. Answer: B

Explanation: Fear or lack of confidence can compromise timely infusion administration during bleeding episodes. The nurse should provide additional education and supervised practice. Emotional readiness is as important as technical skill for home therapy success. Support and reinforcement build caregiver competence.

Subdomain: Transition of Care – Home Education Readiness

Q8. Answer: A

Explanation: Regular survivorship visits focus on growth, development, and screening for late effects. Reviewing immunization status ensures adequate protection after immunosuppressive therapy. Encouraging normal activity promotes psychosocial recovery and resilience. Ongoing education reinforces lifelong health responsibility.

Subdomain: Health Promotion and Maintenance

Q9. Answer: B

Explanation: End-of-life collaboration ensures that all disciplines address physical comfort, emotional support, and family wishes. Shared understanding improves communication and care consistency. Families feel empowered and supported through integrated planning. The approach promotes dignity and quality of life during this stage.

Q10. Answer: C

Explanation: Hospice emphasizes comfort and quality of life rather than cure. The nurse's role is to manage symptoms, facilitate open communication, and provide emotional guidance. Continuing medications that relieve distress supports the family's sense of control. Compassionate presence strengthens trust and eases the transition.

Q11. Answer: B

Explanation: After induction therapy, immunosuppression places the child at high risk for infection. The nurse ensures all caregivers understand signs of fever, hygiene protocols, and when to seek medical help. Coordinating with community nurses provides consistent surveillance. Early intervention prevents severe complications and supports safe recovery at home.

Q12. Answer: A

Explanation: Regular transfusions maintain hemoglobin levels and prevent growth and organ complications. Iron chelation prevents hemosiderosis from repeated transfusions, improving long-term outcomes. Early understanding of this regimen builds family adherence and confidence. Consistent follow-up sustains stability and quality of life.

Subdomain: Health Promotion and Maintenance – Chronic Hematologic Conditions

Q13. Answer: D

Explanation: Following chemotherapy, immune reconstitution may take several months; titers should confirm adequate recovery. Vaccines can then be administered per guidelines to restore full protection. Coordination between oncology and primary care ensures safe timing. This collaborative approach reduces infection risk during reintegration.

Subdomain: Health Promotion and Maintenance – Immunization Review

Q14. Answer: A

Explanation: Clear written plans with contact information enable families to manage symptoms promptly. Providing specific dosing times prevents breakthrough pain and anxiety. Collaboration with palliative services ensures 24-hour access to guidance. This preparation promotes comfort and prevents unnecessary hospital readmissions.

Q15. Answer: A

Explanation: Chemotherapy agents such as doxorubicin and cisplatin can cause long-term cardiac and renal effects. Ongoing surveillance enables early detection and intervention. Including this in the survivorship plan supports lifelong health maintenance. Empowering the adolescent to track follow-ups fosters independence and adherence.

Subdomain: Survivorship – Late Effects Monitoring

Q16. Answer: C

Explanation: Acknowledging anxiety normalizes family feelings and builds trust. Explaining follow-up schedules reassures parents that recurrence will be closely monitored. Open dialogue encourages them to express concerns and seek support early. Emotional validation strengthens coping during survivorship.

Subdomain: Survivorship – Psychological Support

Q17. Answer: A

Explanation: Central line infections are a major risk in pediatric oncology care. Proper hand hygiene and sterile technique during flushing prevent contamination. Teaching and return demonstration confirm caregiver competency. Continuous reinforcement reduces infection-related readmissions and complications.

Subdomain: Transition of Care – Medical Device Education

Q18. Answer: A

Explanation: Written organization systems reduce treatment delays during bleeding episodes. Clear labeling and step-by-step guides improve safety and caregiver confidence. Visual order promotes adherence and reduces stress in emergency situations. Structured preparation supports successful home management.

Subdomain: Transition of Care – Home Preparation

Q19. Answer: D

Explanation: Aligning treatment with family-defined goals maintains respect and compassion. Combining palliative and medical approaches optimizes comfort and hope. Open discussion ensures all team members address physical and emotional needs. This alignment enhances satisfaction and care quality.

Subdomain: End-of-Life Care – Family Goal Integration

Q20. Answer: A

Explanation: Oral chemotherapy requires strict adherence and safety precautions to prevent exposure and dosing errors. The nurse verifies accuracy and demonstrates proper handling and disposal. Teaching ensures understanding of side-effect management and follow-up communication. Comprehensive education supports effective home therapy.
Subdomain: Transition of Care – Medication Safety

Q21. Answer: B

Explanation: Accurate dosing of oral chemotherapy is critical for therapeutic effectiveness and safety. Using a calibrated oral syringe ensures precision and prevents accidental overdose or underdose. Education about handling and disposal enhances family confidence. This step safeguards both patient and caregiver health.
Subdomain: Transition of Care – Medication Safety

Q22. Answer: A

Explanation: Written tools enhance memory and reduce missed visits, which are vital for monitoring chronic conditions. Clear documentation supports family accountability and independence. The nurse ensures parents know how to contact providers for rescheduling or questions. Structured systems increase engagement and treatment continuity.
Subdomain: Transition of Care – Coordination and Follow-up

Q23. Answer: A

Explanation: Self-care development in adolescents with chronic illness promotes autonomy and confidence. Teaching safe infusion practices ensures timely management of bleeding episodes. Encouraging responsibility improves long-term adherence and health outcomes. Transition preparation reduces anxiety and dependency.
Subdomain: Transition of Care – Adolescent Self-Management

Q24. Answer: C

Explanation: Survivorship assessments identify therapy-related late effects that may influence growth and development. Monitoring endocrine and cognitive function helps detect early deficits. Comprehensive evaluation guides appropriate referrals and interventions. This holistic approach promotes lifelong wellness and adaptation.
Subdomain: Survivorship – Late Effects Evaluation

Q25. Answer: A

Explanation: Post-transplant immunosuppression makes infection prevention crucial. Families must understand environmental precautions, including avoiding crowds and maintaining hygiene. Teaching home sanitation and early symptom recognition empowers caregivers. Consistent adherence reduces life-threatening infections.
Subdomain: Transition of Care – Infection Control

Q26. Answer: A

Explanation: Family caregivers often experience physical and emotional strain after prolonged treatment. Linking them to support services provides needed relief and emotional stability. Respite care enhances coping and preserves family functioning. Early recognition prevents caregiver burnout and promotes recovery.
Subdomain: Health Promotion and Maintenance – Family Wellness

Q27. Answer: D

Explanation: Good hygiene and home cleanliness are essential during immune recovery. The nurse reinforces education for all family members and caregivers. Preventive measures like handwashing reduce readmission risk. Coordination ensures all team members reinforce consistent messages.
Subdomain: Transition of Care – Infection Prevention

Q28. Answer: A

Explanation: High altitude and dehydration increase the likelihood of vaso-occlusive crises. Adequate hydration and temperature regulation minimize this risk. Preparing families for environmental triggers promotes safe travel. Education ensures prompt recognition and management of early symptoms.
Subdomain: Health Promotion and Maintenance – Preventive Education

Q29. Answer: A

Explanation: Long-term follow-up identifies delayed complications and secondary malignancies. Regular visits allow healthcare teams to monitor growth, organ function, and psychosocial adjustment. This vigilance maintains health and ensures timely intervention. Survivorship care extends beyond remission.

Subdomain: Survivorship – Family Education

Q30. Answer: B

Explanation: Encouraging honest conversation empowers families to express values and choose care aligned with their beliefs. This shared decision-making enhances emotional comfort and trust. Clear communication allows care to focus on dignity and relief. Compassionate dialogue supports healthy grieving.

Subdomain: End-of-Life Care – Communication and Family Support

Q31. Answer: A

Explanation: Cranial radiation can affect cognition and hormone regulation. Monitoring academic progress and endocrine status detects deficits early. Ongoing collaboration with educators and endocrinologists supports optimal development. Surveillance promotes timely interventions to preserve quality of life.

Subdomain: Survivorship – Neuroendocrine Effects

Q32. Answer: A

Explanation: Introducing the care coordinator facilitates seamless communication between settings. Families benefit from knowing who to contact with concerns. A written contact list prevents confusion and supports proactive care. Early orientation builds trust and continuity.

Subdomain: Transition of Care – Coordination and Communication

Q33. Answer: C

Explanation: Prophylactic therapy maintains factor levels and prevents spontaneous bleeding, preserving joint function. Consistent adherence improves mobility and independence. Early preventive strategies reduce long-term disability. Education reinforces confidence in home management.

Subdomain: Health Promotion and Maintenance – Chronic Illness Prevention

Q34. Answer: A

Explanation: Proper maintenance of central access devices prevents infection and occlusion. Parents must observe for redness, fever, or drainage and seek prompt evaluation. Regular flushing preserves patency. Thorough instruction ensures safety and confidence at home.

Subdomain: Transition of Care – Medical Device Maintenance

Q35. Answer: D

Explanation: A treatment summary provides vital information on prior therapies, potential late effects, and recommended screenings. It ensures continuity of care between oncology and primary providers. Clear documentation prevents duplication and improves long-term monitoring. This promotes cohesive, informed care across settings.

Subdomain: Survivorship – Continuity and Documentation

Q36. Answer: A

Explanation: Siblings often experience confusion, guilt, or isolation during end-of-life care. Encouraging conversation and professional support helps process emotions healthily. Inclusion fosters understanding and family cohesion. Early intervention reduces long-term psychological distress.

Subdomain: End-of-Life Care – Family Dynamics and Support

Q37. Answer: B

Explanation: Leukemic infiltration of the bone marrow suppresses normal erythropoiesis, causing a reduction in red blood cell production. This leads to anemia, reflected by low hemoglobin and hematocrit values. As oxygen-carrying capacity declines, fatigue and pallor become prominent clinical signs.

Subdomain 2A – Pediatric Cancers and Hematologic Disorders

Q38. Answer: B

Explanation: When hemoglobin S becomes deoxygenated, it polymerizes and distorts red cells into a rigid, sickled shape. These cells occlude small vessels and hemolyze early, causing pain and anemia. The recurrent vascular

obstruction leads to chronic organ injury over time.
Subdomain 2A – Pediatric Cancers and Hematologic Disorders

Q39. Answer: C

Explanation: Phase II studies explore how well a treatment works and identify common short-term toxicities. The findings determine whether the therapy should progress to larger comparative trials. Families must understand that participation still involves some uncertainty about benefits.
Subdomain 2B – Clinical Trials

Q40. Answer: B

Explanation: Fanconi anemia results from defective DNA repair, producing chromosomal instability and progressive pancytopenia. Many children present with congenital skeletal or renal anomalies. Diagnosis is confirmed by chromosomal breakage studies and marrow analysis.
Subdomain 2A – Pediatric Cancers and Hematologic Disorders

Q41. Answer: A

Explanation: Methotrexate suppresses bone marrow production, often resulting in thrombocytopenia and increased bleeding risk. Regular platelet monitoring detects early suppression so therapy can be modified. Timely intervention prevents hemorrhagic complications.
Subdomain 2A – Pediatric Cancers and Hematologic Disorders

Q42. Answer: C

Explanation: Autonomy emphasizes the participant's right to make an informed and voluntary decision about research involvement. Transparent discussion of risks and benefits supports respect and trust. Nurses ensure this principle by verifying understanding before enrollment.
Subdomain 2B – Clinical Trials

Q43. Answer: B

Explanation: Repeated transfusions cause accumulation of iron that deposits in vital organs such as the heart, liver, and endocrine glands. Without chelation therapy, this leads to cirrhosis and cardiomyopathy. Ongoing monitoring of ferritin levels guides preventive management.
Subdomain 2A – Pediatric Cancers and Hematologic Disorders

Q44. Answer: B

Explanation: When medication orders conflict, the nurse must withhold administration and clarify the correct order to ensure patient safety. This step demonstrates professional accountability and adherence to practice standards. Clarification prevents medication errors and harm.
Subdomain 2C – Professional Performance

Q45. Answer: C

Explanation: Retinoblastoma involves mutation of the RB1 tumor-suppressor gene, which can be inherited. Familial cases are often bilateral and require genetic screening for siblings. Early detection supports better vision preservation and survival.
Subdomain 2A – Pediatric Cancers and Hematologic Disorders

Q46. Answer: A

Explanation: The scope of practice establishes professional boundaries grounded in licensure laws and national standards. Understanding these boundaries ensures nurses perform duties consistent with their education and role. Adherence protects both patient safety and professional integrity.
Subdomain 2C – Professional Performance

Q47. Answer: B

Explanation: Encouraging the child to select a coping method enhances control and reduces anxiety. This approach aligns with developmental preparation and respects the child's participation in care. Atraumatic care minimizes both physical discomfort and emotional stress.
Subdomain 2C – Professional Performance

Q48. Answer: A

Explanation: A platelet count below $20{,}000/mm^3$ indicates severe thrombocytopenia associated with mucosal bleeding and petechiae. Bone marrow suppression from chemotherapy is a common cause. Platelet transfusions and bleeding precautions are essential interventions.

Subdomain 2A – Pediatric Cancers and Hematologic Disorders

Q49. Answer: B

Explanation: The Oncology Nursing Certification Corporation oversees credentialing for specialty certifications such as CPHON®. It sets eligibility criteria, examination content, and renewal requirements. Certification affirms professional competence in pediatric hematology-oncology nursing.

Subdomain 2C – Professional Performance

Q50. Answer: B

Explanation: Communicating prognosis requires compassionate honesty tailored to the family's readiness to receive information. The nurse supports understanding by clarifying medical details and fostering trust. Sensitive discussion promotes realistic hope and informed decision-making.

Subdomain 2C – Professional Performance

Q51. Answer: D

Explanation: Pain from sickle cell crisis results from blocked blood flow due to sickled red blood cells. Analgesics are necessary to manage pain and improve comfort during the acute crisis. Supportive care, including hydration and oxygen, also aids recovery but pain control is the priority.

Subdomain 2A – Pediatric Cancers and Hematologic Disorders

Q52. Answer: C

Explanation: Cyclophosphamide can cause hemorrhagic cystitis due to the accumulation of acrolein, a toxic metabolite. Adequate hydration and the administration of mesna are key strategies to prevent bladder toxicity. Regular monitoring of urine output and hematuria is critical.

Subdomain 2A – Pediatric Cancers and Hematologic Disorders

Q53. Answer: C

Explanation: Factor replacement therapy is essential for children with hemophilia to prevent bleeding episodes and complications. Proper dosing and adherence to therapy are crucial for maintaining joint and tissue health. Physical activity should be monitored but not completely restricted.

Subdomain 2A – Pediatric Cancers and Hematologic Disorders

Q54. Answer: C

Explanation: Chemotherapy-induced mucositis causes painful mouth sores, and soft, bland foods help reduce irritation. Avoiding acidic or abrasive foods and using non-alcoholic mouthwashes can help alleviate symptoms. Oral care and hydration are key in managing discomfort.

Subdomain 2A – Pediatric Cancers and Hematologic Disorders

Q55. Answer: A

Explanation: Methotrexate can cause nephrotoxicity, especially with high doses or insufficient hydration. Renal function should be closely monitored with regular serum creatinine checks. Adequate hydration and urinary alkalinization help minimize renal damage.

Subdomain 2A – Pediatric Cancers and Hematologic Disorders

Q56. Answer: C

Explanation: Myelodysplastic syndrome (MDS) is characterized by ineffective hematopoiesis and dysplastic changes in the bone marrow. MDS can present with cytopenias, including anemia, and requires close monitoring for transformation into acute leukemia.

Subdomain 2A – Pediatric Cancers and Hematologic Disorders

Q57. Answer: C

Explanation: Prophylactic antibiotics are crucial before stem cell transplantation to prevent infections due to the child's immunocompromised state. In addition to infection prevention, emotional support and comfort measures are important for the child's overall well-being.

Subdomain 2B – Clinical Trials

Q58. Answer: B

Explanation: Blood type and cross-match are essential to ensure compatibility and prevent transfusion reactions. The nurse should verify the patient's blood type and ensure the blood product matches the child's needs. Vital signs should also be monitored during transfusion.

Subdomain 2A – Pediatric Cancers and Hematologic Disorders

Q59. Answer: D

Explanation: Long-term steroid use can lead to increased blood pressure and elevated blood glucose levels. These side effects necessitate monitoring and potential adjustments to diet, activity, and medication. Steroids also increase susceptibility to infections.

Subdomain 2A – Pediatric Cancers and Hematologic Disorders

Q60. Answer: B

Explanation: Retinoblastoma can be inherited through a mutation of the RB1 gene, increasing the risk of secondary cancers, especially osteosarcoma, later in life. Genetic counseling provides important information for family planning and early surveillance for other cancers.

Subdomain 2A – Pediatric Cancers and Hematologic Disorders

Q61. Answer: A

Explanation: Antiemetic medications are critical to managing chemotherapy-induced nausea and vomiting, improving the child's comfort and ability to tolerate treatment. Nutritional support can be adjusted to ensure the child's needs are met while preventing further complications.

Subdomain 3A – Hematology/Oncology Treatment Modalities

Q62. Answer: A

Explanation: Methotrexate can cause mucositis, resulting in painful sores in the mouth and throat. Maintaining oral hygiene, using soft foods, and employing topical agents for pain relief can help manage this side effect.

Subdomain 3A – Hematology/Oncology Treatment Modalities

Q63. Answer: B

Explanation: Survivors of Wilms tumor, especially those treated with radiation, are at increased risk for secondary cancers, such as sarcomas or leukemias, due to the mutagenic effects of radiation therapy. Ongoing surveillance is crucial for early detection.

Subdomain 2A – Pediatric Cancers and Hematologic Disorders

Q64. Answer: B

Explanation: Radiation to the brain can lead to cognitive deficits, particularly in young children, due to the effects on developing brain tissue. Long-term monitoring for developmental milestones and academic progress is important.

Subdomain 3A – Hematology/Oncology Treatment Modalities

Q65. Answer: B

Explanation: Leucovorin is used to "rescue" normal cells from the toxic effects of high-dose methotrexate. It bypasses the block in folate metabolism caused by methotrexate, allowing normal cells to continue DNA synthesis while the cancer cells remain affected.

Subdomain 3A – Hematology/Oncology Treatment Modalities

Q66. Answer: A

Explanation: Radiation therapy for Hodgkin lymphoma, particularly in the neck area, increases the risk of thyroid dysfunction, including hypothyroidism. Lifelong thyroid monitoring is recommended for early detection and management.

Subdomain 3A – Hematology/Oncology Treatment Modalities

Q67. Answer: B

Explanation: Chemotherapy, particularly alkylating agents, increases the risk of secondary malignancies, such as leukemia or lymphoma, years after treatment. Survivors of childhood cancer require long-term monitoring for early detection of new cancers.

Subdomain 3A – Hematology/Oncology Treatment Modalities

Q68. Answer: B

Explanation: A white blood cell count of 1,500/mm^3 indicates neutropenia, which significantly increases the risk of infection. Neutropenic precautions, including isolation and careful monitoring for signs of infection, are essential.

Subdomain 3A – Hematology/Oncology Treatment Modalities

Q69. Answer: B

Explanation: Chemotherapy significantly weakens the immune system, increasing the risk of infections. Parents should be educated about infection prevention strategies, such as proper hand hygiene and avoiding crowds.

Subdomain 3A – Hematology/Oncology Treatment Modalities

Q70. Answer: A

Explanation: Daunorubicin is known for its potential to cause cardiotoxicity, particularly with cumulative dosing. Cardiac function should be regularly monitored with echocardiograms or MUGA scans to detect early signs of damage.

Subdomain 3A – Hematology/Oncology Treatment Modalities

Q71. Answer: B

Explanation: Radiation therapy for Hodgkin lymphoma increases the risk of secondary cancers, particularly after several years of treatment. Survivors must be closely monitored for any signs of secondary malignancies, such as leukemia or solid tumors. Long-term follow-up is essential for early detection.

Subdomain 2A – Pediatric Cancers and Hematologic Disorders

Q72. Answer: C

Explanation: Neutropenia increases the child's risk of infection, making strict hand hygiene and infection control essential. The nurse should implement isolation precautions and monitor for signs of infection. Antibiotic therapy may be needed depending on the child's clinical condition.

Subdomain 2A – Pediatric Cancers and Hematologic Disorders

Q73. Answer: B

Explanation: Ondansetron is a serotonin antagonist commonly used to prevent nausea and vomiting associated with chemotherapy. It works by blocking serotonin receptors in the brain and gastrointestinal tract. This medication is most effective when given before chemotherapy.

Subdomain 2A – Pediatric Cancers and Hematologic Disorders

Q74. Answer: B

Explanation: In the case of joint bleeding, the nurse should elevate the joint and apply ice to reduce swelling and pain. Rest is essential to prevent further damage, and factor replacement therapy should be administered as prescribed.

Subdomain 2A – Pediatric Cancers and Hematologic Disorders

Q75. Answer: C

Explanation: Chemotherapy often leads to mucositis, so gentle brushing and the use of non-alcoholic mouthwash help minimize discomfort and prevent infection. Alcohol-based mouthwashes should be avoided as they can further irritate mucosal tissues.

Subdomain 2A – Pediatric Cancers and Hematologic Disorders

Q76. Answer: B

Explanation: The priority treatment during a vaso-occlusive crisis is pain management and hydration to help improve circulation and prevent further sickling. Transfusions may be necessary later if the crisis does not resolve with supportive care.

Subdomain 2A – Pediatric Cancers and Hematologic Disorders

Q77. Answer: B

Explanation: Methotrexate can cause liver toxicity, so it is essential to monitor liver function tests before starting therapy. Regular monitoring throughout the treatment cycle is necessary to detect any early signs of liver damage.

Subdomain 2A – Pediatric Cancers and Hematologic Disorders

Q78. Answer: D

Explanation: Intrathecal chemotherapy is administered directly into the cerebrospinal fluid to prevent leukemia from spreading to the central nervous system. This is crucial because ALL can often involve the CNS, requiring targeted treatment.

Subdomain 2A – Pediatric Cancers and Hematologic Disorders

Q79. Answer: B

Explanation: Vincristine is a chemotherapy drug that is known for its neurotoxic effects. The most common side effect is peripheral neuropathy, which can cause symptoms such as numbness, tingling, and weakness, especially in the hands and feet.

Subdomain 2A – Pediatric Cancers and Hematologic Disorders

Q80. Answer: B

Explanation: Children with thalassemia often require frequent blood transfusions, leading to

iron overload. The nurse should instruct the family to avoid iron-rich foods and follow the prescribed chelation therapy to manage the excess iron.
Subdomain 2A – Pediatric Cancers and Hematologic Disorders

Q81. Answer: B

Explanation: If an allergic reaction is suspected during a blood transfusion, the first action is to stop the transfusion immediately and notify the provider. The nurse should then assess the child's symptoms and follow institutional protocols for managing transfusion reactions.
Subdomain 2A – Pediatric Cancers and Hematologic Disorders

Q82. Answer: A

Explanation: Graft-versus-host disease (GVHD) occurs when the transplanted immune cells attack the recipient's body. Preventing GVHD is the nurse's priority, and this involves administering immunosuppressive medications and monitoring for signs of immune response.
Subdomain 2A – Pediatric Cancers and Hematologic Disorders

Q83. Answer: B

Explanation: After chemotherapy, the child's immune system is suppressed, making them vulnerable to infections. The nurse should instruct the family to avoid exposure to crowds and anyone who is ill to reduce the risk of infection.
Subdomain 2A – Pediatric Cancers and Hematologic Disorders

Q84. Answer: C

Explanation: Allopurinol is used to prevent kidney damage in children with tumor lysis syndrome by reducing the formation of uric acid crystals. It is essential to monitor kidney function and uric acid levels during therapy.
Subdomain 2A – Pediatric Cancers and Hematologic Disorders

Q85. Answer: B

Explanation: Fatigue is a common symptom in children undergoing leukemia treatment. Encouraging short periods of rest helps the child conserve energy. Additionally, a balanced approach to activity and rest is important for symptom management.
Subdomain 2A – Pediatric Cancers and Hematologic Disorders

Q86. Answer: B

Explanation: A bland, soft diet and regular mouth rinses with saline can help manage the discomfort associated with mucositis. Avoiding spicy, acidic, or hard foods is important to prevent further irritation.
Subdomain 2A – Pediatric Cancers and Hematologic Disorders

Q87. Answer: A

Explanation: During a sickle cell pain crisis, the nurse should prioritize oxygen therapy and pain relief. Adequate hydration and rest are also important to prevent further sickling of red blood cells and reduce pain.
Subdomain 2A – Pediatric Cancers and Hematologic Disorders

Q88. Answer: B

Explanation: Radiation therapy increases the risk of developing secondary cancers, particularly solid tumors or leukemia, years after treatment. Survivors need long-term monitoring to detect any early signs of second malignancies.
Subdomain 2A – Pediatric Cancers and Hematologic Disorders

Q89. Answer: B

Explanation: Factor replacement therapy is critical for children with hemophilia before undergoing any invasive procedure. This ensures that the child has enough clotting factors to prevent bleeding.
Subdomain 2A – Pediatric Cancers and Hematologic Disorders

Q90. Answer: C

Explanation: To prevent infection during neutropenia, the child should be kept away from individuals who are ill, and strict hand hygiene should be followed. The family should also monitor for signs of infection and contact the healthcare provider if any symptoms arise.
Subdomain 2A – Pediatric Cancers and Hematologic Disorders

Q91. Answer: B

Explanation: Methotrexate can cause hepatotoxicity, particularly with high doses. Regular liver function tests are essential to monitor for early signs of liver damage. The nurse should also ensure adequate hydration to support renal function.

Subdomain 2A – Pediatric Cancers and Hematologic Disorders

Q92. Answer: B

Explanation: The primary treatment for a sickle cell crisis is providing adequate hydration and pain relief. This helps alleviate the vaso-occlusive episode by improving circulation and reducing the pain associated with the sickling of red blood cells. Oxygen therapy may be administered if the child is hypoxic.

Subdomain 2A – Pediatric Cancers and Hematologic Disorders

Q93. Answer: D

Explanation: The nurse should immediately stop the infusion and administer epinephrine to treat the anaphylactic reaction. Oxygen therapy and other interventions may follow, but epinephrine is the first line of defense to reverse the symptoms.

Subdomain 2A – Pediatric Cancers and Hematologic Disorders

Q94. Answer: B

Explanation: Providing comfort items such as a toy or blanket can help reduce anxiety by offering the child a sense of security. A calm and reassuring approach is essential to help the child feel supported during the procedure.

Subdomain 2A – Pediatric Cancers and Hematologic Disorders

Q95. Answer: A

Explanation: Vincristine is a chemotherapy agent that can cause constipation and, in severe cases, paralytic ileus. Nurses should monitor the child's bowel function and provide interventions to manage constipation.

Subdomain 2A – Pediatric Cancers and Hematologic Disorders

Q96. Answer: A

Explanation: Frequent blood transfusions can lead to iron overload, which deposits in organs like the liver, heart, and pancreas, potentially causing organ damage. The nurse should monitor iron levels and consider chelation therapy to manage excess iron.

Subdomain 2A – Pediatric Cancers and Hematologic Disorders

Q97. Answer: B

Explanation: The most important intervention for a child with hemophilia is administering factor replacement therapy as prescribed to prevent bleeding episodes. The child can participate in activities with appropriate precautions, but factor therapy is critical for managing the disorder.

Subdomain 2A – Pediatric Cancers and Hematologic Disorders

Q98. Answer: B

Explanation: High-dose corticosteroids commonly cause hyperglycemia and fluid retention. The nurse should monitor blood glucose levels, weight, and for signs of fluid overload. Additionally, these side effects may require adjustments in the child's medication regimen.

Subdomain 2A – Pediatric Cancers and Hematologic Disorders

Q99. Answer: C

Explanation: Induction chemotherapy can cause significant bone marrow suppression, leading to neutropenia. The nurse should closely monitor the white blood cell count and absolute neutrophil count to assess for infection risk and manage neutropenic precautions.

Subdomain 2A – Pediatric Cancers and Hematologic Disorders

Q100. Answer: B

Explanation: Cyclophosphamide is associated with hemorrhagic cystitis due to the accumulation of acrolein, a toxic metabolite. The nurse should ensure adequate hydration and may administer mesna to prevent bladder toxicity.

Subdomain 2A – Pediatric Cancers and Hematologic Disorders

Question (101-200)

Q101. A child is diagnosed with acute leukemia and is receiving vincristine as part of the treatment plan. Which side effect requires the nurse to assess the child for signs of neurotoxicity?

A. Visual disturbances

B. Numbness and tingling in the hands or feet

C. Tachycardia

D. Hypotension

Q102. A child with sickle cell anemia is admitted with a painful crisis. What is the first priority in the nursing management of this child?

A. Administering blood transfusions

B. Administering pain medications and providing hydration

C. Starting intravenous antibiotics

D. Administering oxygen therapy

Q103. A child diagnosed with leukemia is about to start chemotherapy with doxorubicin. What is a major concern associated with this drug?

A. Cardiomyopathy

B. Kidney damage

C. Liver toxicity

D. Ototoxicity

Q104. A nurse is preparing to administer chemotherapy to a child with leukemia. What is the most important consideration before starting treatment?

A. Ensuring the child's growth parameters are within normal limits

B. Verifying that the child has received appropriate immunizations

C. Ensuring the child is well-hydrated and has normal renal function

D. Administering a premedication to prevent allergic reactions

Q105. A nurse is educating a family about managing a child with leukemia who is receiving chemotherapy. Which of the following should be included in the teaching?

A. Encouraging a high-protein, high-calorie diet to support the child's immune system

B. Avoiding all vaccinations during chemotherapy treatment

C. Restricting the child's fluid intake to avoid fluid overload

D. Limiting contact with family members to prevent exposure to infections

Q106. A child with sickle cell disease presents with fever and abdominal pain. What is the most likely diagnosis?

A. Acute splenic sequestration

B. Sickle cell pain crisis

C. Acute chest syndrome

D. Appendicitis

Q107. A child with leukemia is undergoing induction chemotherapy. Which of the following lab results should the nurse monitor closely during this phase of treatment?

A. Hemoglobin and hematocrit levels

B. White blood cell count and absolute neutrophil count

C. Platelet count and iron levels

D. Blood urea nitrogen and creatinine levels

Q108. A child with leukemia is receiving chemotherapy and experiences a sudden increase in blood pressure. What is the most likely cause of this symptom?

A. Dehydration from vomiting

B. Adrenal insufficiency due to steroid use

C. Fluid overload from IV fluids

D. Infiltration of the chemotherapy drug

Q109. A child receiving chemotherapy for leukemia is at risk for developing anemia. What should the nurse monitor closely in this child?

A. Hemoglobin and hematocrit levels

B. Serum calcium and phosphate levels

C. Blood glucose levels

D. Electrolyte balance

Q110. A child is receiving chemotherapy with doxorubicin. What is the most important intervention to prevent cardiotoxicity from this drug?

A. Monitoring blood pressure and heart rate

B. Administering diuretics to reduce fluid retention

C. Regularly assessing cardiac function with echocardiograms or MUGA scans

D. Encouraging exercise to improve circulation

Q111. A child with leukemia is receiving radiation therapy to the chest area. What is the most significant long-term concern associated with this treatment?

A. Development of second cancers, particularly breast cancer
B. Cardiomyopathy and heart failure
C. Hearing loss and tinnitus
D. Chronic renal failure

Q112. A child is receiving chemotherapy for leukemia and develops mucositis. Which intervention is most helpful in managing this condition?
A. Administering antacids for acid reflux
B. Encouraging the child to avoid all foods and liquids
C. Providing soft, bland foods and frequent mouth rinses
D. Applying ice packs to the affected areas

Q113. A child with sickle cell disease presents with severe pain and swelling in the joints. What is the nurse's first intervention?
A. Administering pain medications and fluids
B. Applying cold compresses to the joints
C. Encouraging the child to rest the affected limb
D. Preparing the child for surgery to drain the joint

Q114. A child undergoing chemotherapy is at risk for neutropenia. What is the most important measure to prevent infection in this child?
A. Administering prophylactic antibiotics
B. Placing the child in a private room and using strict hand hygiene
C. Encouraging physical activity to improve circulation
D. Restricting fluid intake to prevent overhydration

Q115. A nurse is caring for a child who has been newly diagnosed with leukemia. Which of the following is the most important for the nurse to assess during the initial evaluation?
A. Nutritional status and caloric intake
B. Psychosocial impact on the family
C. Presence of fever or infection
D. Understanding of the treatment regimen

Q116. A nurse is preparing a child with leukemia for a bone marrow biopsy. Which action should the nurse take to reduce the child's anxiety?
A. Allow the child to choose the position for the procedure
B. Provide detailed explanations of the procedure to the child and family
C. Encourage the child to remain silent during the procedure
D. Administer a sedative prior to the procedure

Q117. A child with leukemia is receiving methotrexate therapy. What is the most important nursing consideration during this treatment?
A. Monitoring for signs of infection
B. Ensuring adequate hydration and monitoring kidney function
C. Monitoring blood glucose levels regularly
D. Administering vitamin supplements as prescribed

Q118. A child with sickle cell disease is receiving a blood transfusion. The nurse should closely monitor for signs of which potential complication?
A. Allergic reaction
B. Cardiac arrhythmias
C. Graft-versus-host disease
D. Iron overload

Q119. A child with leukemia is undergoing induction chemotherapy. Which lab result is most indicative of bone marrow suppression during this phase of treatment?
A. Increased white blood cell count
B. Low hemoglobin and hematocrit levels
C. Elevated platelet count
D. Increased reticulocyte count

Q120. A child is receiving radiation therapy for brain cancer. What is a common long-term effect of this treatment in children?
A. Growth and development delays
B. Hair loss and scalp infections
C. Hearing loss and tinnitus
D. Chronic respiratory issues

Q121. A nurse is caring for a child with leukemia who is receiving high-dose corticosteroids. What is the most important potential side effect to monitor for?
A. Gastrointestinal bleeding
B. Hyperglycemia and fluid retention
C. Bone marrow suppression
D. Cardiac arrhythmias

Q122. A nurse is caring for a child with leukemia who is receiving vincristine therapy. What is a common side effect of this drug?
A. Hypertension
B. Nephrotoxicity
C. Peripheral neuropathy
D. Cardiotoxicity
Q123. A nurse is providing education to the parents of a child with hemophilia. What is the most important instruction for the nurse to provide?
A. Administer factor replacement therapy regularly to prevent bleeding episodes
B. Avoid all physical activity to prevent joint damage
C. Ensure that the child does not receive any immunizations
D. Encourage the child to participate in high-impact sports
Q124. A child with leukemia is experiencing fatigue as a side effect of chemotherapy. What is the best intervention to help manage this symptom?
A. Encourage high-energy activities to improve stamina
B. Provide frequent rest periods throughout the day
C. Limit fluid intake to reduce fatigue
D. Administer stimulant medications to combat tiredness
Q125. A nurse is caring for a child who is undergoing chemotherapy and develops mouth sores. Which intervention should the nurse prioritize?
A. Encouraging the child to drink acidic beverages to numb the pain
B. Administering a pain-relieving mouth rinse
C. Restricting the child's oral intake to prevent further irritation
D. Providing a high-calorie diet to promote healing
Q126. A child with leukemia is receiving vincristine as part of the treatment regimen. What side effect is most commonly associated with this drug?
A. Peripheral neuropathy
B. Hyperglycemia
C. Ototoxicity
D. Pulmonary fibrosis
Q127. A child with thalassemia requires frequent blood transfusions. What is the nurse's primary concern in the long term?
A. Iron overload
B. Risk of stroke
C. Development of secondary cancers
D. Bone marrow failure
Q128. A nurse is caring for a child who is receiving chemotherapy with cyclophosphamide. Which side effect should the nurse be most concerned about?
A. Nephrotoxicity
B. Hypertension
C. Hemorrhagic cystitis
D. Cardiotoxicity
Q129. A child with leukemia is receiving radiation therapy to the brain. What is a potential long-term effect of this treatment?
A. Cognitive impairments and learning disabilities
B. Chronic kidney disease
C. Hearing loss
D. Growth delays and short stature
Q130. A nurse is preparing a child with leukemia for a lumbar puncture. Which action is essential to reduce the child's anxiety?
A. Allowing the child to choose a comfort item, such as a blanket or toy
B. Encouraging the child to remain silent during the procedure
C. Administering sedatives to induce sleep
D. Avoiding all discussion about the procedure
Q131. A nurse is caring for a child with leukemia who is receiving high-dose chemotherapy. What is the priority intervention to prevent infection during neutropenia?
A. Administering broad-spectrum antibiotics
B. Providing a low-bacteria diet
C. Implementing strict hand hygiene and isolation precautions
D. Encouraging physical activity to improve circulation
Q132. A nurse is assessing a child with leukemia who is receiving methotrexate. Which lab result is most concerning in this child?
A. Platelet count of 150,000/mm^3
B. Hemoglobin level of 11 g/dL

C. Serum creatinine level of 1.5 mg/dL
D. White blood cell count of 30,000/mm^3

Q133. A child with sickle cell disease presents with pain and swelling in the joints. What is the nurse's priority action?
A. Administering opioids for pain relief
B. Applying heat to the affected joints
C. Increasing the child's fluid intake
D. Encouraging the child to rest the affected joints

Q134. A child with leukemia is receiving high-dose corticosteroids. What is the nurse's primary concern with this treatment?
A. Increased risk of infection
B. Gastrointestinal bleeding
C. Hyperglycemia and fluid retention
D. Ototoxicity

Q135. A child with leukemia is receiving chemotherapy with cyclophosphamide. What is the nurse's primary concern regarding this medication?
A. Hemorrhagic cystitis
B. Ototoxicity
C. Nephrotoxicity
D. Cardiotoxicity

Q136. A child with leukemia is undergoing radiation therapy. What is a common long-term effect of this treatment?
A. Growth hormone deficiency
B. Neurological deficits
C. Cardiovascular complications
D. Hearing loss

Q137. A child with a history of leukemia is receiving a blood transfusion. What is the most important action the nurse should take before the transfusion?
A. Give the child an antihistamine to prevent an allergic reaction
B. Administer pain medication to prevent discomfort
C. Monitor the child's temperature and vital signs
D. Ensure the child's blood type is matched with the donor blood

Q138. A nurse is caring for a child undergoing chemotherapy with vincristine. What is the most common side effect associated with this drug?
A. Peripheral neuropathy
B. Hyperkalemia
C. Bone marrow suppression
D. Pulmonary toxicity

Q139. A child receiving methotrexate for leukemia is at risk for developing mucositis. What is the most effective intervention to manage this side effect?
A. Provide frequent mouth rinses with salt water or baking soda solution
B. Administer a high-protein diet to promote tissue healing
C. Encourage the child to use an alcohol-based mouthwash
D. Restrict the child's food intake to avoid further irritation

Q140. A nurse is educating the parents of a child with leukemia about the side effects of chemotherapy. What is the most important side effect to discuss regarding the use of high-dose steroids?
A. Increased risk of infection
B. Gastrointestinal bleeding
C. Hyperglycemia and fluid retention
D. Ototoxicity

Q141. A child with leukemia is receiving chemotherapy that includes anthracyclines. What is the primary concern related to this drug class?
A. Cardiotoxicity
B. Hepatotoxicity
C. Renal toxicity
D. Neutropenia

Q142. A child with leukemia is experiencing hair loss due to chemotherapy. What is the best way to help the child cope with this side effect?
A. Encourage the child to wear a wig or hat if desired
B. Explain that hair loss will be permanent
C. Recommend cutting the hair short to make the transition easier
D. Avoid discussing the hair loss with the child

Q143. A child with leukemia is receiving chemotherapy that includes methotrexate. Which side effect should the nurse monitor for during therapy?
A. Hypoglycemia
B. Alopecia

C. Mucositis and nausea
D. Hyperkalemia

Q144. A child with leukemia is receiving chemotherapy with doxorubicin. Which of the following is the most important monitoring parameter for this drug?
A. Liver function tests
B. Cardiac function (e.g., echocardiogram or MUGA scan)
C. Blood glucose levels
D. Urine output and renal function

Q145. A nurse is educating the parents of a child with sickle cell anemia about pain management during a vaso-occlusive crisis. What is the most important intervention?
A. Administering pain medications and ensuring hydration
B. Encouraging physical activity to prevent clotting
C. Providing a low-sodium diet to reduce swelling
D. Applying cold compresses to the painful areas

Q146. A nurse is caring for a child with leukemia who is receiving methotrexate. What is the primary concern regarding this medication?
A. Hepatotoxicity
B. Nephrotoxicity
C. Neurotoxicity
D. Ototoxicity

Q147. A child with leukemia is receiving vincristine as part of their chemotherapy regimen. What is the most common side effect associated with vincristine?
A. Peripheral neuropathy
B. Alopecia
C. Neutropenia
D. Hemorrhagic cystitis

Q148. A nurse is providing care to a child receiving chemotherapy with doxorubicin. Which assessment is most important to monitor for potential adverse effects of this drug?
A. Cardiac function (e.g., echocardiogram or MUGA scan)
B. Liver function tests
C. Renal function tests
D. Blood glucose levels

Q149. A child with leukemia is undergoing chemotherapy and is at high risk for infection. What is the most important intervention to reduce this risk?
A. Administering broad-spectrum antibiotics
B. Placing the child in reverse isolation
C. Administering anti-fungal therapy
D. Encouraging physical activity to improve circulation

Q150. A child with sickle cell disease is experiencing a painful vaso-occlusive crisis. What is the nurse's primary focus in managing this crisis?
A. Administering blood transfusions
B. Providing pain relief and hydration
C. Administering antibiotics for infection
D. Encouraging ambulation to relieve pain

Q151. A child with leukemia is receiving high-dose corticosteroids as part of their treatment regimen. What is a common side effect of corticosteroids that the nurse should monitor for?
A. Hyperglycemia
B. Hypotension
C. Weight loss
D. Decreased white blood cell count

Q152. A nurse is educating the parents of a child with thalassemia who is receiving regular blood transfusions. What is the most important long-term concern related to this treatment?
A. Iron overload
B. Vitamin D deficiency
C. Bone fractures
D. Liver failure

Q153. A nurse is caring for a child receiving chemotherapy with cyclophosphamide. Which side effect should the nurse be most concerned about?
A. Nephrotoxicity
B. Pulmonary fibrosis
C. Hemorrhagic cystitis
D. Ototoxicity

Q154. A nurse is caring for a child with leukemia who is receiving methotrexate therapy. What is the most important action to reduce the risk of methotrexate toxicity?
A. Administering leucovorin as prescribed
B. Providing a high-protein diet
C. Limiting fluid intake
D. Monitoring blood glucose levels

Q155. A child with leukemia is experiencing nausea and vomiting after receiving chemotherapy. What is the most effective intervention to manage this side effect?
A. Administering antiemetic medications before chemotherapy
B. Encouraging the child to drink large amounts of fluids
C. Providing high-calorie, high-fat snacks
D. Restricting the child's oral intake to reduce vomiting

Q156. A child with leukemia is receiving radiation therapy to the brain. What is the most common long-term effect of this treatment in children?
A. Hearing loss
B. Cognitive and developmental delays
C. Bone fractures
D. Gastrointestinal complications

Q157. A nurse is caring for a child with leukemia who is experiencing bone pain due to chemotherapy. What is the most appropriate intervention to manage this pain?
A. Administering acetaminophen as needed
B. Encouraging non-pharmacologic pain relief methods, such as guided imagery
C. Providing opioid analgesics as prescribed
D. Applying cold packs to the affected areas

Q158. A child with leukemia is receiving chemotherapy with etoposide. What is a potential side effect of this medication that the nurse should monitor for?
A. Ototoxicity
B. Myelosuppression
C. Hyperkalemia
D. Liver toxicity

Q159. A nurse is caring for a child with leukemia who is receiving methotrexate. What is the most important nursing consideration when administering this drug?
A. Ensuring that the child is well-hydrated
B. Limiting the child's intake of vitamin C
C. Administering a corticosteroid prior to the chemotherapy
D. Monitoring for signs of dehydration

Q160. A nurse is providing education to the parents of a child with sickle cell anemia. Which of the following is the most important instruction regarding pain management during a crisis?
A. Administering opioids as needed for pain relief
B. Encouraging physical activity to reduce clotting
C. Limiting fluid intake to reduce swelling
D. Applying cold compresses to painful areas

Q161. A child with leukemia is receiving high-dose chemotherapy. What is the most important side effect the nurse should monitor for during treatment?
A. Hypertension
B. Bone marrow suppression
C. Hyperglycemia
D. Gastrointestinal bleeding

Q162. A child with leukemia is receiving radiation therapy to the brain. What is the most common long-term effect of this treatment?
A. Cognitive and developmental delays
B. Hearing loss
C. Gastrointestinal complications
D. Bone fractures

Q163. A child with leukemia is receiving chemotherapy with doxorubicin. What is the most important nursing consideration regarding this drug?
A. Monitoring for nephrotoxicity
B. Monitoring for signs of cardiotoxicity
C. Administering leucovorin as prescribed
D. Monitoring for myelosuppression

Q164. A child with leukemia is receiving chemotherapy with methotrexate. What is the most common side effect of methotrexate that the nurse should monitor for?
A. Mucositis
B. Nephrotoxicity
C. Hepatotoxicity
D. Neuropathy

Q165. A child with leukemia is receiving chemotherapy with vincristine. What is the most common side effect associated with vincristine therapy?
A. Peripheral neuropathy
B. Neutropenia
C. Cardiotoxicity
D. Pulmonary fibrosis

Q166. A child with leukemia is receiving chemotherapy that includes methotrexate. Which of the following is the most important side effect to monitor for during therapy?
A. Mucositis
B. Alopecia
C. Nephrotoxicity
D. Hearing loss

Q167. A child with sickle cell anemia is admitted with a painful crisis. What is the priority action for the nurse?
A. Administering pain medications and fluids
B. Administering oxygen therapy
C. Providing blood transfusions
D. Encouraging ambulation to improve circulation

Q168. A child with leukemia is receiving chemotherapy and develops neutropenia. What should the nurse prioritize in the care of this child?
A. Administering blood products as needed
B. Providing reverse isolation to prevent infection
C. Increasing physical activity to improve circulation
D. Encouraging high-protein foods to promote healing

Q169. A nurse is educating the parents of a child with leukemia who is receiving chemotherapy. What is the most important instruction regarding infection prevention?
A. Avoid administering any over-the-counter medications
B. Keep the child away from crowds and sick individuals
C. Ensure the child avoids all physical activity
D. Limit the child's fluid intake to reduce swelling

Q170. A child with leukemia is receiving high-dose corticosteroids. What is a common side effect of these medications that the nurse should monitor for?
A. Dehydration and electrolyte imbalances
B. Weight gain and fluid retention
C. Hypoglycemia
D. Bone marrow suppression

Q171. A nurse is caring for a child with leukemia who is receiving chemotherapy with vincristine. What is the most common side effect associated with this drug?
A. Peripheral neuropathy
B. Cardiotoxicity
C. Myelosuppression
D. Gastrointestinal bleeding

Q172. A child with leukemia is undergoing radiation therapy to the brain. What is a common long-term effect of this treatment?
A. Cognitive and developmental delays
B. Hearing loss
C. Cardiovascular complications
D. Bone fractures

Q173. A child with leukemia is receiving chemotherapy with doxorubicin. What is the primary concern with this medication?
A. Ototoxicity
B. Hepatotoxicity
C. Cardiotoxicity
D. Nephrotoxicity

Q174. A nurse is educating the family of a child receiving chemotherapy. What is the most important advice to prevent mucositis?
A. Use a hard-bristled toothbrush to remove plaque
B. Rinse the mouth with alcohol-based mouthwash
C. Provide frequent mouth rinses with saline or baking soda solution
D. Encourage the child to avoid all oral intake during chemotherapy

Q175. A child with sickle cell anemia is experiencing a pain crisis. What is the nurse's first priority in managing this crisis?
A. Administering blood transfusions
B. Providing pain relief and fluids
C. Administering antibiotics
D. Increasing oxygen levels with a mask

Q176. A child with leukemia is receiving high-dose chemotherapy. What is the nurse's priority intervention to manage the side effects of this treatment?
A. Administering medications to manage nausea and vomiting
B. Monitoring vital signs for signs of shock
C. Providing a high-protein diet to promote healing

D. Encouraging physical activity to prevent muscle wasting

Q177. A nurse is caring for a child who is receiving chemotherapy with cyclophosphamide. Which of the following is a key nursing intervention to prevent a common side effect?

A. Administering mesna to prevent hemorrhagic cystitis
B. Limiting fluid intake to reduce fluid retention
C. Administering antibiotics to prevent infections
D. Monitoring blood glucose levels

Q178. A nurse is educating the family of a child receiving chemotherapy about preventing infection. What should the nurse recommend?

A. Keep the child in isolation at all times
B. Avoid all vaccines during chemotherapy treatment
C. Monitor for signs of infection and seek prompt medical attention
D. Limit the child's fluid intake to reduce swelling

Q179. A child with leukemia is receiving chemotherapy and develops fatigue. What is the most appropriate action for the nurse to take?

A. Encourage the child to engage in vigorous physical activity
B. Administer stimulant medications to reduce fatigue
C. Provide frequent rest periods throughout the day
D. Limit the child's fluid intake to conserve energy

Q180. A nurse is caring for a child receiving chemotherapy with methotrexate. What is the most important action to minimize side effects from this medication?

A. Administer leucovorin as prescribed
B. Provide a high-calcium diet
C. Limit fluid intake to prevent edema
D. Monitor blood glucose levels regularly

Q181. A child diagnosed with leukemia is undergoing chemotherapy with cyclophosphamide. What is the most important side effect of this drug that the nurse should monitor for?

A. Nephrotoxicity
B. Hemorrhagic cystitis
C. Cardiotoxicity
D. Hyperkalemia

Q182. A child with leukemia is receiving methotrexate. What is the most important nursing consideration to reduce the risk of toxicity?

A. Administer leucovorin as prescribed
B. Provide a low-protein diet
C. Encourage high-sodium foods
D. Limit fluid intake to prevent edema

Q183. A child receiving chemotherapy for leukemia develops neutropenia. What is the most important intervention for the nurse to implement?

A. Administering antifungal medications
B. Providing a high-calorie diet
C. Administering broad-spectrum antibiotics
D. Implementing reverse isolation and strict hand hygiene

Q184. A child with leukemia is receiving vincristine as part of their chemotherapy regimen. What is the most common side effect of vincristine?

A. Bone marrow suppression
B. Peripheral neuropathy
C. Ototoxicity
D. Alopecia

Q185. A nurse is caring for a child with leukemia who is receiving radiation therapy to the brain. What is the most common long-term side effect of this treatment in children?

A. Cognitive and developmental delays
B. Hearing loss
C. Cardiomyopathy
D. Growth hormone deficiency

Q186. A child with leukemia is undergoing chemotherapy. Which of the following is the most significant side effect of high-dose corticosteroids?

A. Hypoglycemia
B. Weight gain and fluid retention
C. Hypertension
D. Osteoporosis

Q187. A nurse is educating the parents of a child with leukemia about the side effects of chemotherapy. What is the most common side effect the nurse should prepare the parents for?

A. Nausea and vomiting

B. Alopecia
C. Bone marrow suppression
D. Mucositis

Q188. A child with sickle cell disease is in the hospital for a pain crisis. What is the first priority for the nurse?
A. Administering opioid pain medications
B. Providing oxygen therapy
C. Starting a blood transfusion
D. Increasing oral fluid intake

Q189. A child with leukemia is receiving chemotherapy with etoposide. What side effect is most commonly associated with this medication?
A. Hemorrhagic cystitis
B. Nephrotoxicity
C. Ototoxicity
D. Myelosuppression

Q190. A child with leukemia is receiving chemotherapy with doxorubicin. What is the most important nursing consideration during treatment with this drug?
A. Monitoring for signs of cardiac toxicity
B. Monitoring for signs of nephrotoxicity
C. Monitoring for signs of liver toxicity
D. Monitoring for signs of hyperkalemia

Q191. A child with leukemia is receiving chemotherapy and is at risk for developing mucositis. Which intervention is most appropriate?
A. Administering antifungal medications
B. Encouraging the child to use a soft-bristled toothbrush
C. Providing a high-fiber diet
D. Encouraging the child to avoid all oral intake

Q192. A nurse is caring for a child with leukemia who is receiving high-dose chemotherapy. What is the priority nursing intervention during the nadir phase of chemotherapy?
A. Monitoring vital signs for signs of shock
B. Administering blood products as prescribed
C. Providing pain relief and hydration
D. Preventing infection through strict hygiene and isolation

Q193. A nurse is caring for a child with leukemia who is receiving methotrexate therapy. What is the primary concern associated with this drug?
A. Hepatotoxicity
B. Mucositis and nausea
C. Bone marrow suppression
D. Ototoxicity

Q194. A child with leukemia is receiving high-dose chemotherapy. What is the most common side effect that the nurse should monitor for during chemotherapy?
A. Cardiac arrhythmias
B. Bone marrow suppression
C. Renal failure
D. Gastrointestinal bleeding

Q195. A nurse is caring for a child with leukemia receiving chemotherapy with cyclophosphamide. What is the priority action to prevent a common side effect of this medication?
A. Administer mesna to prevent hemorrhagic cystitis
B. Monitor renal function closely
C. Provide a high-calorie diet
D. Administer antifungal medications to prevent infections

Q196. A nurse is educating the parents of a child with leukemia about the side effects of chemotherapy. Which of the following should the nurse emphasize?
A. The child may experience hair loss
B. The child will not be able to eat solid foods during treatment
C. The child should avoid all physical activity during therapy
D. The child is at increased risk for infections

Q197. A child with leukemia is receiving chemotherapy with cyclophosphamide. What is the most important nursing consideration for this drug?
A. Monitoring for hemorrhagic cystitis
B. Monitoring for hepatotoxicity
C. Monitoring for signs of nephrotoxicity
D. Ensuring adequate hydration to prevent dehydration

Q198. A child with leukemia is receiving high-dose corticosteroids. What is a common side effect of steroid therapy in children?
A. Weight loss and anorexia
B. Fluid retention and weight gain
C. Hypercalcemia
D. Bone marrow suppression

Q199. A child with leukemia is receiving chemotherapy. What is the nurse's primary concern during the nadir phase of chemotherapy?

A. Bone marrow suppression

B. Infection

C. Nausea and vomiting

D. Gastrointestinal bleeding

Q200. A child with sickle cell disease is experiencing a pain crisis. What is the first priority in the management of this condition?

A. Administering blood transfusions

B. Providing pain relief and hydration

C. Administering antibiotics

D. Initiating oxygen therapy

Answer Key and Explanation (101-200)

Q101. Answer: B

Explanation: Vincristine can cause peripheral neuropathy, which manifests as numbness and tingling in the hands or feet. The nurse should monitor for these signs and report any changes in neurological status to the healthcare provider.

Subdomain 2A – Pediatric Cancers and Hematologic Disorders

Q102. Answer: B

Explanation: The primary treatment for a painful sickle cell crisis is providing pain relief and hydration to help reduce the sickling of red blood cells and improve circulation. Oxygen therapy and blood transfusions may be needed if the crisis does not resolve.

Subdomain 2A – Pediatric Cancers and Hematologic Disorders

Q103. Answer: A

Explanation: Doxorubicin is known to cause cardiomyopathy and heart failure, especially with cumulative doses. The nurse should monitor the child's cardiac function closely, using echocardiograms or MUGA scans to detect any early signs of heart damage.

Subdomain 2A – Pediatric Cancers and Hematologic Disorders

Q104. Answer: C

Explanation: Before administering chemotherapy, it is important to ensure that the child is well-hydrated and has normal renal function to help prevent renal toxicity from certain chemotherapeutic agents.

Subdomain 2A – Pediatric Cancers and Hematologic Disorders

Q105. Answer: A

Explanation: A high-protein, high-calorie diet helps support the child's nutritional needs during chemotherapy, especially since treatment can cause nausea and reduced appetite. Good nutrition is important for maintaining strength and immune function.

Subdomain 2A – Pediatric Cancers and Hematologic Disorders

Q106. Answer: A

Explanation: Acute splenic sequestration occurs when sickled red blood cells block blood flow to the spleen, causing it to enlarge and potentially leading to a life-threatening drop in hemoglobin. This condition requires immediate medical attention.

Subdomain 2A – Pediatric Cancers and Hematologic Disorders

Q107. Answer: B

Explanation: Induction chemotherapy causes significant bone marrow suppression, which results in neutropenia and thrombocytopenia. The nurse should monitor the white blood cell count and absolute neutrophil count to assess infection risk.

Subdomain 2A – Pediatric Cancers and Hematologic Disorders

Q108. Answer: B

Explanation: Steroid medications, commonly used in leukemia treatment, can cause fluid retention and hypertension. The nurse should monitor the child's blood pressure closely and report significant increases.

Subdomain 2A – Pediatric Cancers and Hematologic Disorders

Q109. Answer: A

Explanation: Chemotherapy can suppress bone marrow function, leading to decreased red blood cell production and anemia. The nurse should monitor hemoglobin and hematocrit levels to assess the child's oxygen-carrying capacity.

Subdomain 2A – Pediatric Cancers and Hematologic Disorders

Q110. Answer: C

Explanation: Doxorubicin is known to cause cardiotoxicity, so regular cardiac function assessments, such as echocardiograms or MUGA scans, are essential to detect early signs of heart damage and prevent long-term complications.

Subdomain 2A – Pediatric Cancers and Hematologic Disorders

Q111. Answer: A

Explanation: Radiation therapy to the chest area increases the risk of developing second cancers, especially breast cancer, years after treatment. Survivors of childhood leukemia should be monitored regularly for early detection of secondary malignancies.

Subdomain 2A – Pediatric Cancers and Hematologic Disorders

Q112. Answer: C

Explanation: Mucositis is a common side effect of chemotherapy, and providing soft, bland foods and frequent mouth rinses with a saline solution can reduce irritation and promote healing. Avoiding acidic, spicy, or hot foods is essential to minimize discomfort.

Subdomain 2A – Pediatric Cancers and Hematologic Disorders

Q113. Answer: A

Explanation: Pain management and hydration are the primary interventions during a sickle cell crisis. Hydration helps reduce the viscosity of blood and alleviates pain, while pain relief allows the child to rest and recover. Cold compresses may be used, but the priority is pain and hydration.

Subdomain 2A – Pediatric Cancers and Hematologic Disorders

Q114. Answer: B

Explanation: Neutropenic precautions, including placing the child in a private room and practicing strict hand hygiene, are essential to prevent infections. The child should also avoid exposure to sick individuals, and a low-bacteria diet may be recommended.

Subdomain 2A – Pediatric Cancers and Hematologic Disorders

Q115. Answer: C

Explanation: Fever and infection are common complications in children with leukemia due to bone marrow suppression and immune system dysfunction. Early identification and treatment of infections are critical to prevent life-threatening complications.

Subdomain 2A – Pediatric Cancers and Hematologic Disorders

Q116. Answer: B

Explanation: Explaining the procedure in age-appropriate terms helps reduce anxiety by preparing the child and family for what to expect. Offering emotional support and addressing any fears or concerns is essential to alleviate stress.

Subdomain 2A – Pediatric Cancers and Hematologic Disorders

Q117. Answer: B

Explanation: Methotrexate can cause nephrotoxicity, so it is important to monitor kidney function and ensure the child is well-hydrated to help prevent kidney damage. Hydration also helps promote excretion of the drug and its metabolites.

Subdomain 2A – Pediatric Cancers and Hematologic Disorders

Q118. Answer: D

Explanation: Blood transfusions can lead to iron overload, which can damage organs such as the heart, liver, and pancreas. The nurse should monitor iron levels and provide chelation therapy if necessary to prevent organ damage.

Subdomain 2A – Pediatric Cancers and Hematologic Disorders

Q119. Answer: B

Explanation: Induction chemotherapy often causes bone marrow suppression, leading to decreased red blood cell production. This results in low hemoglobin and hematocrit levels, which may cause fatigue and pallor in the child.

Subdomain 2A – Pediatric Cancers and Hematologic Disorders

Q120. Answer: A

Explanation: Radiation therapy to the brain can impact growth and development, particularly in young children. It can affect cognitive function, hormone production, and physical growth, making long-term monitoring essential.

Subdomain 2A – Pediatric Cancers and Hematologic Disorders

Q121. Answer: B

Explanation: High-dose corticosteroids are known to cause hyperglycemia and fluid retention. The nurse should monitor blood glucose levels and the child's weight, as these side effects can lead to other complications if left unaddressed.

Subdomain 2A – Pediatric Cancers and Hematologic Disorders

Q122. Answer: C

Explanation: Vincristine is known to cause peripheral neuropathy, leading to symptoms such as numbness and tingling in the hands or feet. The nurse should monitor for these signs

and report any changes in the child's neurological status.
Subdomain 2A – Pediatric Cancers and Hematologic Disorders

Q123. Answer: A

Explanation: Administering factor replacement therapy is essential to prevent bleeding episodes and maintain joint health in children with hemophilia. The child can participate in non-contact sports with appropriate precautions, but factor therapy is crucial.
Subdomain 2A – Pediatric Cancers and Hematologic Disorders

Q124. Answer: B

Explanation: Fatigue is a common side effect of chemotherapy. Frequent rest periods throughout the day help conserve energy and manage this symptom effectively. The child should be encouraged to maintain a balanced activity level without overexertion.
Subdomain 2A – Pediatric Cancers and Hematologic Disorders

Q125. Answer: B

Explanation: Pain-relieving mouth rinses, such as those containing salt or baking soda, can help manage the discomfort caused by chemotherapy-induced mucositis. The child should also be encouraged to avoid acidic, spicy, and hot foods to minimize irritation.
Subdomain 2A – Pediatric Cancers and Hematologic Disorders

Q126. Answer: A

Explanation: Vincristine is associated with peripheral neuropathy, which can cause symptoms such as numbness, tingling, and weakness, especially in the hands and feet. The nurse should monitor for these symptoms and report any changes.
Subdomain 2A – Pediatric Cancers and Hematologic Disorders

Q127. Answer: A

Explanation: Frequent blood transfusions lead to iron overload, which can deposit in organs such as the liver, heart, and pancreas. The nurse should monitor iron levels and provide chelation therapy to prevent organ damage.
Subdomain 2A – Pediatric Cancers and Hematologic Disorders

Q128. Answer: C

Explanation: Cyclophosphamide can cause hemorrhagic cystitis, a condition in which blood appears in the urine. The nurse should ensure adequate hydration and administer mesna, if prescribed, to reduce the risk of bladder toxicity.
Subdomain 2A – Pediatric Cancers and Hematologic Disorders

Q129. Answer: A

Explanation: Radiation therapy to the brain can cause cognitive impairments and learning disabilities, particularly in younger children. Long-term monitoring and educational support are essential for children who have received brain radiation.
Subdomain 2A – Pediatric Cancers and Hematologic Disorders

Q130. Answer: A

Explanation: Allowing the child to choose a comfort item, such as a blanket or toy, can help reduce anxiety by providing a sense of security. Age-appropriate explanations and reassurance are also important to alleviate fear.
Subdomain 2A – Pediatric Cancers and Hematologic Disorders

Q131. Answer: C

Explanation: Strict hand hygiene and isolation precautions are essential to prevent infection in children with neutropenia. The nurse should also ensure that the child avoids exposure to sick individuals and implements a low-bacteria diet.
Subdomain 2A – Pediatric Cancers and Hematologic Disorders

Q132. Answer: C

Explanation: Methotrexate can cause nephrotoxicity, so an elevated serum creatinine level is concerning. The nurse should monitor kidney function closely and ensure the child is well-hydrated to prevent renal damage.
Subdomain 2A – Pediatric Cancers and Hematologic Disorders

Q133. Answer: C

Explanation: Hydration is essential in managing sickle cell crisis, as it helps to reduce the viscosity of blood and prevent further sickling of red blood cells. Pain relief and rest are also important, but hydration is the priority.

Subdomain 2A – Pediatric Cancers and Hematologic Disorders

Q134. Answer: C

Explanation: High-dose corticosteroids can cause hyperglycemia and fluid retention, which can lead to complications such as edema and increased blood pressure. The nurse should monitor blood glucose levels and the child's weight closely.

Subdomain 2A – Pediatric Cancers and Hematologic Disorders

Q135. Answer: A

Explanation: Cyclophosphamide is associated with hemorrhagic cystitis, a condition that causes blood in the urine due to the toxic metabolite acrolein. The nurse should ensure the child is well-hydrated and monitor urine output for early signs of this complication.

Subdomain 3A – Hematology/Oncology Treatment Modalities

Q136. Answer: A

Explanation: Radiation therapy can impact the hypothalamic-pituitary axis, leading to growth hormone deficiency, especially in younger children. Long-term follow-up is necessary to monitor for this and other endocrine abnormalities.

Subdomain 3A – Hematology/Oncology Treatment Modalities

Q137. Answer: D

Explanation: Ensuring that the child's blood type is properly matched with the donor blood is crucial to prevent transfusion reactions. The nurse should also monitor vital signs during the transfusion and be prepared to respond to any reactions.

Subdomain 3A – Hematology/Oncology Treatment Modalities

Q138. Answer: A

Explanation: Vincristine is known for causing peripheral neuropathy, which can lead to numbness, tingling, and weakness, particularly in the hands and feet. The nurse should assess the child for these symptoms and report any changes.

Subdomain 3A – Hematology/Oncology Treatment Modalities

Q139. Answer: A

Explanation: Mucositis can be effectively managed by providing frequent mouth rinses with salt water or baking soda solution, which helps to soothe the mouth and reduce irritation. The child should also avoid alcohol-based mouthwashes, which can exacerbate irritation.

Subdomain 3A – Hematology/Oncology Treatment Modalities

Q140. Answer: C

Explanation: High-dose steroids can cause hyperglycemia and fluid retention. The nurse should educate the parents about monitoring for these side effects, including changes in the child's weight and blood glucose levels, and report any significant changes to the healthcare provider.

Subdomain 3A – Hematology/Oncology Treatment Modalities

Q141. Answer: A

Explanation: Anthracyclines, such as doxorubicin, are known for their potential to cause cardiotoxicity, especially with cumulative dosing. The nurse should monitor the child's cardiac function with echocardiograms or MUGA scans to detect early signs of heart damage.

Subdomain 3A – Hematology/Oncology Treatment Modalities

Q142. Answer: A

Explanation: Hair loss is a common side effect of chemotherapy, and the best way to help the child cope is to encourage them to wear a wig, hat, or scarf if they wish. It's important to support the child's choices and help them feel in control of the situation.

Subdomain 3A – Hematology/Oncology Treatment Modalities

Q143. Answer: C

Explanation: Mucositis and nausea are common side effects of methotrexate therapy. The nurse should assess the child for these symptoms and provide supportive care, such as antiemetics and mouth rinses, to alleviate discomfort.

Subdomain 3A – Hematology/Oncology Treatment Modalities

Q144. Answer: B

Explanation: Doxorubicin is known for its potential to cause cardiotoxicity, so monitoring cardiac function, including echocardiograms or

MUGA scans, is essential. Early detection of heart damage can help guide dose adjustments and prevent permanent damage.
Subdomain 3A – Hematology/Oncology Treatment Modalities

Q145. Answer: A

Explanation: Pain management and hydration are the primary interventions during a vaso-occlusive crisis in sickle cell anemia. Adequate hydration helps improve blood flow and reduce sickling of red blood cells, while pain medications alleviate discomfort.
Subdomain 3A – Hematology/Oncology Treatment Modalities

Q146. Answer: B

Explanation: Methotrexate can cause nephrotoxicity, especially at high doses. The nurse should monitor renal function closely, ensuring that the child is well-hydrated to minimize renal damage and facilitate the elimination of the drug.
Subdomain 3A – Hematology/Oncology Treatment Modalities

Q147. Answer: A

Explanation: Vincristine is known to cause peripheral neuropathy, which can result in numbness, tingling, and weakness, especially in the hands and feet. The nurse should monitor the child for these symptoms and provide supportive care as needed.
Subdomain 3A – Hematology/Oncology Treatment Modalities

Q148. Answer: A

Explanation: Doxorubicin is known for its potential to cause cardiotoxicity, and it is critical to monitor the child's cardiac function, such as through echocardiograms or MUGA scans. Early detection of heart damage can prevent long-term complications.
Subdomain 3A – Hematology/Oncology Treatment Modalities

Q149. Answer: B

Explanation: Placing the child in reverse isolation is essential to protect them from infections due to neutropenia and immunosuppression from chemotherapy. Strict hand hygiene and avoiding contact with sick individuals are also key components of infection prevention.
Subdomain 3A – Hematology/Oncology Treatment Modalities

Q150. Answer: B

Explanation: During a sickle cell crisis, the primary focus is pain management and hydration. Hydration helps reduce the viscosity of blood and prevent further sickling of red blood cells. Pain relief is also essential to improve the child's comfort.
Subdomain 3A – Hematology/Oncology Treatment Modalities

Q151. Answer: A

Explanation: High-dose corticosteroids can cause hyperglycemia due to their effects on glucose metabolism. The nurse should monitor blood glucose levels regularly and report any significant increases to the healthcare provider.
Subdomain 3A – Hematology/Oncology Treatment Modalities

Q152. Answer: A

Explanation: Regular blood transfusions can lead to iron overload, which can damage organs such as the heart, liver, and pancreas. The nurse should educate the parents about monitoring iron levels and providing chelation therapy to manage excess iron.
Subdomain 3A – Hematology/Oncology Treatment Modalities

Q153. Answer: C

Explanation: Cyclophosphamide is associated with hemorrhagic cystitis, a condition in which blood appears in the urine. The nurse should ensure adequate hydration and may administer mesna to prevent this complication.
Subdomain 3A – Hematology/Oncology Treatment Modalities

Q154. Answer: A

Explanation: Leucovorin is administered to "rescue" normal cells from the toxic effects of methotrexate by bypassing the blockage of folate metabolism. The nurse should ensure the child receives leucovorin as prescribed to prevent methotrexate toxicity.
Subdomain 3A – Hematology/Oncology Treatment Modalities

Q155. Answer: A

Explanation: Administering antiemetic medications before chemotherapy can help

prevent nausea and vomiting. Preemptive antiemetics are most effective in controlling chemotherapy-induced nausea and vomiting.
Subdomain 3A – Hematology/Oncology Treatment Modalities

Q156. Answer: B

Explanation: Radiation therapy to the brain can affect cognitive function, leading to developmental delays, particularly in younger children. Long-term monitoring and educational support are important for children who have received brain radiation.
Subdomain 3A – Hematology/Oncology Treatment Modalities

Q157. Answer: C

Explanation: For moderate to severe pain caused by chemotherapy, opioid analgesics are often necessary for effective pain management. The nurse should assess pain levels regularly and administer medications as prescribed.
Subdomain 3A – Hematology/Oncology Treatment Modalities

Q158. Answer: B

Explanation: Etoposide can cause myelosuppression, leading to decreased blood cell counts, including white blood cells, red blood cells, and platelets. The nurse should monitor complete blood counts (CBC) regularly and manage complications such as infection or bleeding.
Subdomain 3A – Hematology/Oncology Treatment Modalities

Q159. Answer: A

Explanation: Methotrexate is nephrotoxic, and adequate hydration is essential to help prevent renal damage and facilitate the excretion of the drug. The nurse should monitor the child's fluid intake and urine output closely.
Subdomain 3A – Hematology/Oncology Treatment Modalities

Q160. Answer: A

Explanation: During a sickle cell crisis, pain management with opioids is essential to provide relief and improve the child's comfort. Hydration and rest are also important, but pain relief is the top priority.
Subdomain 3A – Hematology/Oncology Treatment Modalities

Q161. Answer: B

Explanation: High-dose chemotherapy is known to cause bone marrow suppression, leading to neutropenia, anemia, and thrombocytopenia. The nurse should monitor blood counts closely and be prepared to manage complications such as infections and bleeding.
Subdomain 3A – Hematology/Oncology Treatment Modalities

Q162. Answer: A

Explanation: Radiation therapy to the brain, especially in younger children, can lead to cognitive and developmental delays. Long-term follow-up is necessary to monitor the child's intellectual and developmental progress.
Subdomain 3A – Hematology/Oncology Treatment Modalities

Q163. Answer: B

Explanation: Doxorubicin is known to cause cardiotoxicity, so it is essential to monitor the child's cardiac function through echocardiograms or MUGA scans. Early detection of cardiac damage can help prevent long-term complications.
Subdomain 3A – Hematology/Oncology Treatment Modalities

Q164. Answer: A

Explanation: Methotrexate often causes mucositis, which results in painful sores in the mouth and gastrointestinal tract. The nurse should monitor for these symptoms and provide supportive care such as mouth rinses and pain relief.
Subdomain 3A – Hematology/Oncology Treatment Modalities

Q165. Answer: A

Explanation: Vincristine is associated with peripheral neuropathy, leading to symptoms such as numbness and tingling in the hands and feet. The nurse should monitor for these symptoms and intervene as needed.
Subdomain 3A – Hematology/Oncology Treatment Modalities

Q166. Answer: C

Explanation: Methotrexate can cause nephrotoxicity, especially at high doses. The nurse should monitor renal function closely, ensuring adequate hydration and monitoring

urine output to minimize the risk of renal damage.
Subdomain 3A – Hematology/Oncology Treatment Modalities

Q167. Answer: A

Explanation: The priority during a sickle cell pain crisis is providing pain relief and ensuring adequate hydration to reduce blood viscosity. Pain management helps reduce the sickling of red blood cells, and hydration improves circulation.
Subdomain 3A – Hematology/Oncology Treatment Modalities

Q168. Answer: B

Explanation: Neutropenic precautions, including reverse isolation, are essential to protect the child from infections due to a suppressed immune system. Strict hand hygiene and limiting exposure to sick individuals are also crucial.
Subdomain 3A – Hematology/Oncology Treatment Modalities

Q169. Answer: B

Explanation: During chemotherapy, the child's immune system is suppressed, so it is essential to avoid exposure to sick individuals and large crowds to reduce the risk of infections. Good hygiene practices and proper vaccination are also important.
Subdomain 3A – Hematology/Oncology Treatment Modalities

Q170. Answer: B

Explanation: High-dose corticosteroids can cause weight gain and fluid retention due to their effects on sodium and fluid balance. The nurse should monitor the child's weight, blood pressure, and electrolytes regularly during steroid therapy.
Subdomain 3A – Hematology/Oncology Treatment Modalities

Q171. Answer: A

Explanation: Vincristine is associated with peripheral neuropathy, which can cause numbness, tingling, and weakness, particularly in the hands and feet. The nurse should monitor for these symptoms and adjust care accordingly.
Subdomain 3A – Hematology/Oncology Treatment Modalities

Q172. Answer: A

Explanation: Radiation therapy to the brain can cause cognitive and developmental delays, particularly in younger children. These effects can impact learning and intellectual development, necessitating long-term follow-up and support.
Subdomain 3A – Hematology/Oncology Treatment Modalities

Q173. Answer: C

Explanation: Doxorubicin is known for its potential to cause cardiotoxicity, which can lead to heart failure with cumulative doses. The nurse should monitor the child's cardiac function closely using echocardiograms or MUGA scans.
Subdomain 3A – Hematology/Oncology Treatment Modalities

Q174. Answer: C

Explanation: Frequent mouth rinses with saline or baking soda solution help manage the discomfort of mucositis, a common side effect of chemotherapy. The nurse should also advise avoiding alcohol-based mouthwashes and encourage soft, bland foods.
Subdomain 3A – Hematology/Oncology Treatment Modalities

Q175. Answer: B

Explanation: Pain relief and hydration are the primary interventions during a sickle cell pain crisis. Pain relief helps reduce the suffering caused by vaso-occlusion, and fluids help reduce blood viscosity and improve circulation.
Subdomain 3A – Hematology/Oncology Treatment Modalities

Q176. Answer: A

Explanation: High-dose chemotherapy often causes nausea and vomiting, so the nurse should prioritize administering antiemetics before and after treatment to reduce these side effects. Maintaining hydration and nutritional support is also important.
Subdomain 3A – Hematology/Oncology Treatment Modalities

Q177. Answer: A

Explanation: Cyclophosphamide can cause hemorrhagic cystitis due to a toxic metabolite. Administering mesna and ensuring adequate hydration can help prevent this side effect by

neutralizing the metabolite and promoting urinary excretion.
Subdomain 3A – Hematology/Oncology Treatment Modalities

Q178. Answer: C

Explanation: The child's immune system is suppressed during chemotherapy, so it is essential to monitor for signs of infection, such as fever, and seek prompt medical attention if symptoms arise. Preventive measures such as good hygiene and avoiding sick individuals are also important.
Subdomain 3A – Hematology/Oncology Treatment Modalities

Q179. Answer: C

Explanation: Fatigue is a common side effect of chemotherapy, and the best way to manage it is by providing frequent rest periods to conserve energy. A balance of activity and rest is important to prevent overexertion.
Subdomain 3A – Hematology/Oncology Treatment Modalities

Q180. Answer: A

Explanation: Leucovorin is administered to "rescue" normal cells from the toxic effects of methotrexate. It helps to prevent methotrexate toxicity by bypassing the blockage of folate metabolism, allowing normal cells to continue functioning.
Subdomain 3A – Hematology/Oncology Treatment Modalities

Q181. Answer: B

Explanation: Cyclophosphamide is associated with hemorrhagic cystitis, a condition caused by the toxic metabolite acrolein. The nurse should ensure adequate hydration and may administer mesna to help prevent this complication.
Subdomain 3A – Hematology/Oncology Treatment Modalities

Q182. Answer: A

Explanation: Leucovorin is used to "rescue" normal cells from the toxic effects of methotrexate by bypassing the block in folate metabolism. It helps to protect healthy cells and minimize side effects.
Subdomain 3A – Hematology/Oncology Treatment Modalities

Q183. Answer: D

Explanation: Neutropenic precautions, including reverse isolation and strict hand hygiene, are essential to protect the child from infections due to suppressed immunity. Monitoring for signs of infection is also crucial.
Subdomain 3A – Hematology/Oncology Treatment Modalities

Q184. Answer: B

Explanation: Vincristine commonly causes peripheral neuropathy, which can lead to symptoms such as numbness, tingling, and weakness in the hands and feet. Monitoring and early intervention can help manage these symptoms.
Subdomain 3A – Hematology/Oncology Treatment Modalities

Q185. Answer: A

Explanation: Radiation therapy to the brain, particularly in young children, can cause cognitive and developmental delays. Long-term follow-up with neurodevelopmental assessments is essential to address any issues early.
Subdomain 3A – Hematology/Oncology Treatment Modalities

Q186. Answer: B

Explanation: High-dose corticosteroids often lead to weight gain and fluid retention, as well as increased appetite. The nurse should monitor the child's weight and blood pressure regularly during steroid therapy.
Subdomain 3A – Hematology/Oncology Treatment Modalities

Q187. Answer: A

Explanation: Nausea and vomiting are common side effects of chemotherapy. The nurse should educate the parents about antiemetic medications and dietary modifications to help manage these symptoms.
Subdomain 3A – Hematology/Oncology Treatment Modalities

Q188. Answer: A

Explanation: Pain relief is the priority during a sickle cell crisis. Opioid analgesics are commonly used to manage moderate to severe pain. Hydration and oxygen therapy may also be necessary but pain relief should be addressed first.

Subdomain 3A – Hematology/Oncology Treatment Modalities

Q189. Answer: D

Explanation: Etoposide is known to cause myelosuppression, which results in decreased blood cell production. The nurse should monitor the child's blood counts closely and manage any complications, such as infection or bleeding.

Subdomain 3A – Hematology/Oncology Treatment Modalities

Q190. Answer: A

Explanation: Doxorubicin is known for its potential to cause cardiotoxicity, so the nurse should monitor cardiac function through regular assessments, such as echocardiograms or MUGA scans, to detect early signs of damage.

Subdomain 3A – Hematology/Oncology Treatment Modalities

Q191. Answer: B

Explanation: A soft-bristled toothbrush and gentle oral care are essential for managing mucositis, a common side effect of chemotherapy. The nurse should also recommend frequent mouth rinses with saline or baking soda solution to reduce discomfort.

Subdomain 3A – Hematology/Oncology Treatment Modalities

Q192. Answer: D

Explanation: During the nadir phase of chemotherapy, when the white blood cell count is at its lowest, infection prevention is the priority. The nurse should implement strict hand hygiene and isolation precautions to reduce the risk of infection.

Subdomain 3A – Hematology/Oncology Treatment Modalities

Q193. Answer: B

Explanation: Methotrexate commonly causes mucositis and nausea as side effects. The nurse should provide supportive care, such as antiemetics and mouth rinses, to alleviate discomfort.

Subdomain 3A – Hematology/Oncology Treatment Modalities

Q194. Answer: B

Explanation: Bone marrow suppression is a common side effect of high-dose chemotherapy, leading to neutropenia, anemia, and thrombocytopenia. The nurse should monitor blood counts regularly and be prepared to manage complications such as infection and bleeding.

Subdomain 3A – Hematology/Oncology Treatment Modalities

Q195. Answer: A

Explanation: Cyclophosphamide is known to cause hemorrhagic cystitis, so mesna is administered to prevent this side effect. The nurse should also ensure adequate hydration and monitor urine output for signs of toxicity.

Subdomain 3A – Hematology/Oncology Treatment Modalities

Q196. Answer: D

Explanation: Chemotherapy can suppress the immune system, putting the child at an increased risk for infections. The nurse should emphasize the importance of infection prevention, including hand hygiene and avoiding exposure to sick individuals.

Subdomain 3A – Hematology/Oncology Treatment Modalities

Q197. Answer: A

Explanation: Cyclophosphamide can cause hemorrhagic cystitis due to its toxic metabolite acrolein. The nurse should ensure that the child is adequately hydrated and may administer mesna as prescribed to reduce the risk of bladder toxicity.

Subdomain 3A – Hematology/Oncology Treatment Modalities

Q198. Answer: B

Explanation: High-dose corticosteroids can cause fluid retention and weight gain. The nurse should monitor the child's weight and blood pressure and educate the family about these potential side effects.

Subdomain 3A – Hematology/Oncology Treatment Modalities

Q199. Answer: B

Explanation: During the nadir phase, when the child's white blood cell count is at its lowest, the risk for infection is highest. The nurse should implement strict infection control precautions and monitor for signs of infection.

Subdomain 3A – Hematology/Oncology Treatment Modalities

Q200. Answer: B

Explanation: Pain relief and hydration are the primary interventions during a sickle cell pain crisis. Pain relief helps reduce the suffering caused by vaso-occlusion, and hydration helps improve circulation and reduce blood viscosity.

Subdomain 3A – Hematology/Oncology Treatment Modalities

Question (201-300)

Q201. A child receiving cisplatin for osteosarcoma reports ringing in the ears. Which nursing action is most appropriate?

A. Encourage hydration

B. Notify the provider for potential ototoxicity

C. Administer antiemetic therapy

D. Schedule audiometric evaluation after therapy completion

Q202. A patient receiving interferon therapy for relapsed neuroblastoma complains of fatigue and flu-like symptoms. Which intervention should the nurse anticipate?

A. Discontinue treatment immediately

B. Administer acetaminophen before doses

C. Reduce fluid intake

D. Initiate antibiotic prophylaxis

Q203. A child undergoing CAR-T cell therapy develops fever, hypotension, and hypoxia. What condition should the nurse suspect?

A. Cytokine release syndrome

B. Tumor lysis syndrome

C. Disseminated intravascular coagulation

D. Sepsis

Q204. A child receiving methotrexate has an absolute neutrophil count of $400/mm^3$. Which teaching should the nurse provide to the family?

A. Encourage school attendance

B. Avoid crowds and sick contacts

C. Limit oral fluid intake

D. Continue all routine immunizations

Q205. A child undergoing cranial radiation develops somnolence and irritability three weeks after treatment. What is the most likely cause?

A. Tumor recurrence

B. Radiation-induced somnolence syndrome

C. Hypothyroidism

D. Increased intracranial pressure

Q206. A child receiving doxorubicin presents with fatigue and shortness of breath. Which diagnostic test is most appropriate?

A. Chest X-ray

B. Echocardiogram

C. Pulmonary function test

D. Electroencephalogram

Q207. A patient with leukemia receiving cytarabine develops ataxia and confusion. What should the nurse suspect?

A. Cerebellar toxicity

B. Seizure disorder

C. Meningeal relapse

D. Hypoglycemia

Q208. During administration of vincristine, the child reports burning and pain at the IV site. What is the nurse's immediate action?

A. Apply warm compresses

B. Stop the infusion immediately

C. Flush with saline

D. Elevate the affected limb

Q209. A nurse caring for a child post–stem cell transplant notes oral mucositis with ulcerations and pain. What is the best nursing intervention?

A. Encourage mouth rinses with normal saline

B. Provide lemon-glycerin swabs

C. Withhold oral care to prevent bleeding

D. Use alcohol-based mouthwash

Q210. A patient receiving etoposide experiences sudden hypotension during infusion. What should the nurse do first?

A. Stop the infusion

B. Administer an antihistamine

C. Slow the infusion rate

D. Notify the provider after completion

Q211. A child is to receive cyclophosphamide. What prophylactic measure should the nurse implement to prevent hemorrhagic cystitis?

A. Administer mesna and increase hydration

B. Limit oral fluids

C. Provide antiemetics

D. Monitor neurologic status

Q212. A patient receiving total body irradiation (TBI) before stem cell transplant develops erythema and dry desquamation. What is the best nursing action?

A. Apply petroleum-based ointments

B. Use gentle cleansing with mild soap and water

C. Expose the area to sunlight

D. Apply ice packs to the affected area

Q213. Following hematopoietic stem cell transplant, a child develops jaundice, weight gain, and hepatomegaly. Which complication is suspected?

A. Hepatic veno-occlusive disease
B. Graft-versus-host disease
C. Tumor lysis syndrome
D. Acute pancreatitis

Q214. A nurse caring for a patient receiving bleomycin notes shortness of breath and crackles. What should the nurse do?
A. Hold further doses and notify the provider
B. Encourage deep breathing exercises
C. Continue treatment and document findings
D. Administer furosemide for fluid overload

Q215. A child undergoing chemotherapy reports tingling in the fingers and difficulty buttoning clothes. Which effect is suspected?
A. Nephrotoxicity
B. Myelosuppression
C. Peripheral neuropathy
D. Ototoxicity

Q216. During biotherapy administration, the nurse observes urticaria and wheezing. What is the immediate nursing action?
A. Stop the infusion and maintain airway
B. Continue the infusion at a slower rate
C. Administer oral antihistamine
D. Notify pharmacy for a new bag

Q217. A child is receiving G-CSF following chemotherapy. What is the expected therapeutic effect?
A. Reduction in platelet count
B. Increased neutrophil recovery
C. Decreased hemoglobin production
D. Prevention of nausea and vomiting

Q218. A nurse is preparing to administer intrathecal chemotherapy. Which safety precaution is essential?
A. Verify route and drug label with another chemotherapy-certified nurse
B. Flush the line before and after administration
C. Administer concurrently with IV chemotherapy
D. Dilute the drug with normal saline

Q219. A patient undergoing chemotherapy presents with oral ulcers and white patches on the tongue. What is the likely cause?
A. Fungal infection secondary to immunosuppression
B. Viral reactivation
C. Poor oral hygiene
D. Nutritional deficiency

Q220. After hematopoietic stem cell transplant, the patient develops skin rash, diarrhea, and elevated liver enzymes. What condition should the nurse suspect?
A. Acute graft-versus-host disease
B. Veno-occlusive disease
C. Sepsis
D. Tumor lysis syndrome

Q221. A nurse is preparing a child to receive intrathecal methotrexate. Which nursing action is most important prior to the procedure?
A. Administer antiemetic medication
B. Ensure the patient has been premedicated with corticosteroids
C. Verify the drug, dose, and route with another chemotherapy-certified nurse
D. Confirm that hydration is adequate

Q222. A patient receiving busulfan as part of a transplant conditioning regimen reports headaches and blurred vision. The nurse suspects which complication?
A. Hypertension
B. Seizure activity
C. Hepatic veno-occlusive disease
D. Tumor lysis syndrome

Q223. A nurse caring for a child after hematopoietic stem cell transplant observes watery diarrhea and an erythematous rash on the palms and soles. What is the likely cause?
A. Cytomegalovirus colitis
B. Acute graft-versus-host disease
C. Irritable bowel syndrome
D. Bacterial enteritis

Q224. A patient receiving bleomycin develops a new cough and fine crackles on auscultation. Which test should the nurse anticipate?
A. Pulmonary function tests
B. Abdominal ultrasound
C. Echocardiogram
D. Brain MRI

Q225. A nurse is monitoring a child receiving doxorubicin for signs of cardiotoxicity. Which clinical finding would be most concerning?
A. Bradycardia
B. Peripheral neuropathy
C. Dyspnea on exertion
D. Decreased appetite

Q226. A child receiving vincristine reports difficulty walking and decreased ankle reflexes. Which nursing intervention is most appropriate?
A. Encourage ambulation as tolerated
B. Report findings for possible dose adjustment
C. Apply heat to the affected areas
D. Provide a low-protein diet
Q227. A nurse observes that a child receiving cytarabine has developed fever and conjunctivitis. What action should the nurse take?
A. Administer corticosteroid eye drops as prescribed
B. Apply warm compresses
C. Stop the chemotherapy immediately
D. Encourage increased fluid intake
Q228. A child receiving total body irradiation prior to transplant experiences nausea and vomiting. Which nursing intervention is most effective for symptom control?
A. Encourage small, frequent meals
B. Administer prescribed antiemetic before each session
C. Offer clear liquids only
D. Provide deep breathing exercises
Q229. A nurse caring for a patient receiving monoclonal antibody therapy notes fever and chills shortly after infusion starts. What is the nurse's immediate action?
A. Stop the infusion and assess the patient
B. Continue infusion at the same rate
C. Administer antibiotic therapy
D. Notify the provider after infusion completion
Q230. A child receiving high-dose methotrexate therapy is prescribed leucovorin rescue. What is the purpose of this medication?
A. Prevent nephrotoxicity
B. Reduce nausea and vomiting
C. Protect normal cells from methotrexate toxicity
D. Enhance the cytotoxic effect of methotrexate
Q231. A nurse notes petechiae and prolonged bleeding in a child undergoing chemotherapy. Which lab result is most likely abnormal?
A. Hemoglobin
B. Platelet count
C. Sodium level
D. White blood cell count
Q232. A child receiving chemotherapy reports painful urination and blood in the urine. Which nursing action takes priority?
A. Encourage oral fluids
B. Collect a urine culture
C. Notify the provider immediately
D. Provide warm sitz baths
Q233. Following stem cell infusion, a child develops fever, dyspnea, and pulmonary infiltrates. What should the nurse suspect?
A. Engraftment syndrome
B. Bacterial pneumonia
C. Fluid overload
D. Viral bronchitis
Q234. A patient undergoing chemotherapy complains of tingling in the hands and feet. Which medication is most associated with this symptom?
A. Etoposide
B. Methotrexate
C. Cyclophosphamide
D. Vincristine
Q235. A child receiving biotherapy experiences hypotension and tachycardia during infusion. What should the nurse do first?
A. Stop the infusion and assess vital signs
B. Place the child in Trendelenburg position
C. Administer corticosteroids
D. Notify the pharmacy
Q236. A patient receiving radiation therapy for abdominal lymphoma reports diarrhea and cramping. Which dietary advice should the nurse provide?
A. Increase fiber intake
B. Consume low-lactose, low-residue foods
C. Increase intake of raw fruits and vegetables
D. Avoid all carbohydrates
Q237. A nurse caring for a child after hematopoietic stem cell transplant observes a generalized erythematous rash and elevated bilirubin levels. What complication is suspected?
A. Graft-versus-host disease
B. Sinusoidal obstruction syndrome
C. Allergic drug reaction
D. Viral exanthem

Q238. During chemotherapy administration, the nurse notes erythema and swelling at the IV site. Which immediate action is required?
A. Stop the infusion and assess for extravasation
B. Apply heat to the affected site
C. Continue the infusion slowly
D. Flush the IV line with saline
Q239. A nurse provides education to parents of a child starting cyclophosphamide therapy. Which instruction is most important?
A. Avoid citrus beverages
B. Restrict oral fluids before bedtime
C. Use acetaminophen for nausea
D. Encourage frequent voiding and fluid intake
Q240. A child receiving stem cell transplant develops elevated bilirubin, hepatomegaly, and ascites. Which intervention is most appropriate?
A. Restrict fluids and monitor weight closely
B. Encourage increased salt intake
C. Administer growth factors
D. Provide high-protein diet
Q241. A child with acute lymphoblastic leukemia develops hematuria during ifosfamide therapy. Which nursing action is the priority?
A. Increase oral fluid intake
B. Notify the provider immediately
C. Provide pain medication
D. Encourage bed rest
Q242. A child receiving cisplatin complains of persistent nausea despite antiemetics. What additional intervention is most appropriate?
A. Offer bland foods and frequent small meals
B. Increase IV fluid rate
C. Administer a second antiemetic from a different class
D. Stop the chemotherapy infusion
Q243. A nurse is caring for a child undergoing CAR-T cell therapy who suddenly develops confusion and expressive aphasia. What should the nurse suspect?
A. Tumor lysis syndrome
B. Intracranial hemorrhage
C. Immune effector cell-associated neurotoxicity
D. Seizure disorder
Q244. A child undergoing total body irradiation reports dry, peeling skin. Which nursing action is most appropriate?
A. Apply gentle, fragrance-free moisturizer
B. Use alcohol wipes for cleansing
C. Encourage daily exfoliation
D. Cover the area with adhesive dressings
Q245. A child receiving doxorubicin asks why heart function tests are needed. What is the best explanation by the nurse?
A. "The tests monitor for infection caused by chemotherapy."
B. "They ensure your heart remains strong while receiving treatment."
C. "They check if the medication affects your kidney function."
D. "The tests measure how well you tolerate the medication's side effects."
Q246. A patient with leukemia is receiving filgrastim (G-CSF). Which assessment finding requires immediate nursing action?
A. Bone pain in the lower back
B. Fever of 101°F (38.3°C)
C. Mild fatigue
D. Increased white blood cell count
Q247. A child receiving methotrexate develops elevated creatinine levels. What should the nurse anticipate?
A. Decrease in hydration rate
B. Discontinuation of folic acid supplements
C. Initiation of antibiotics
D. Increase in leucovorin rescue dosing
Q248. A child receiving biotherapy experiences chills and rigors during infusion. Which medication is likely administered to manage this reaction?
A. Epinephrine
B. Diphenhydramine
C. Lorazepam
D. Morphine
Q249. A patient receiving high-dose cytarabine develops slurred speech and unsteady gait. What should the nurse do first?
A. Stop chemotherapy and notify the provider
B. Administer antiemetic therapy
C. Monitor fluid balance closely
D. Encourage the patient to rest

Q250. A child receiving etoposide develops hypotension during infusion. What is the appropriate nursing intervention?
A. Stop the infusion and monitor vital signs
B. Increase the infusion rate
C. Administer corticosteroids
D. Flush the IV line with saline

Q251. A nurse provides teaching to parents of a child receiving cyclophosphamide. Which statement indicates correct understanding?
A. "We'll limit bathroom trips during the night."
B. "We should give fewer fluids before bedtime."
C. "We'll stop fluids if there's any vomiting."
D. "We will make sure our child drinks plenty of fluids."

Q252. A child with neuroblastoma receives isotretinoin as maintenance therapy. Which side effect should the nurse monitor for?
A. Dry skin and lips
B. Alopecia
C. Constipation
D. Myelosuppression

Q253. A patient receiving hematopoietic stem cell transplant develops jaundice and rapid weight gain. Which complication should the nurse suspect?
A. Acute GVHD
B. Hepatic sinusoidal obstruction syndrome
C. Sepsis
D. Engraftment syndrome

Q254. During radiation therapy, a child develops a sore mouth with difficulty eating. Which intervention should the nurse recommend?
A. Use soft, bland foods and saline mouth rinses
B. Provide citrus juices between meals
C. Offer spicy foods to stimulate appetite
D. Encourage brushing with alcohol-based mouthwash

Q255. A nurse observes redness and swelling at the chemotherapy IV site. What should be done first?
A. Stop the infusion and assess the site
B. Elevate the limb and continue the infusion
C. Apply heat to promote absorption
D. Flush the IV with saline

Q256. A child receiving cyclophosphamide develops burning on urination. Which lab finding is expected?
A. Leukocytosis
B. Elevated bilirubin
C. Low potassium
D. Hematuria

Q257. A nurse caring for a child on methotrexate therapy reviews the medication list and identifies a potential interaction with:
A. Trimethoprim-sulfamethoxazole
B. Ondansetron
C. Diphenhydramine
D. Acetaminophen

Q258. A child undergoing biotherapy reports severe fatigue and mild depression. Which nursing intervention is appropriate?
A. Encourage rest and provide emotional support
B. Stop therapy immediately
C. Administer corticosteroids
D. Increase oral hydration

Q259. A nurse monitors a child after stem cell transplant for early signs of infection. Which finding is most concerning?
A. Poor appetite
B. Fatigue
C. Temperature of 38.1°C (100.6°F)
D. Alopecia

Q260. A patient receiving radiation to the abdomen reports nausea before each session. Which strategy best reduces anticipatory symptoms?
A. Relaxation techniques and antiemetic before treatment
B. Increasing fiber intake
C. Avoiding eating for 8 hours prior
D. Switching to a liquid-only diet

Q261. A nurse caring for a child receiving ifosfamide notes new-onset confusion and lethargy. Which complication should the nurse suspect?
A. Hepatic failure
B. Metabolic alkalosis
C. Encephalopathy
D. Sepsis

Q262. A patient receiving high-dose methotrexate develops mouth ulcers and a sore throat. Which action is most important?

A. Begin antibiotic prophylaxis
B. Increase leucovorin rescue
C. Encourage cold beverages
D. Provide oral antihistamines

Q263. A child undergoing hematopoietic stem cell transplantation develops a pruritic, erythematous rash and diarrhea 20 days post-transplant. Which condition is most likely?

A. Sinusoidal obstruction syndrome
B. Acute graft-versus-host disease
C. Drug-induced dermatitis
D. Engraftment syndrome

Q264. A patient receiving bleomycin reports shortness of breath and a nonproductive cough. What diagnostic test should the nurse anticipate?

A. Pulmonary function testing
B. Electrocardiogram
C. Abdominal ultrasound
D. Brain MRI

Q265. A child receiving cyclophosphamide exhibits dark, bloody urine. Which medication should the nurse expect to administer?

A. Mesna
B. Leucovorin
C. Filgrastim
D. Ondansetron

Q266. A nurse is caring for a patient who develops erythema and swelling during doxorubicin infusion. What is the immediate nursing action?

A. Apply warm compresses
B. Stop the infusion and assess for extravasation
C. Administer corticosteroids
D. Flush the IV line with saline

Q267. A nurse provides discharge instructions for a child receiving oral retinoid therapy for neuroblastoma. Which statement indicates correct understanding?

A. "We will use sunscreen daily to prevent skin irritation."
B. "We should avoid giving the medication with food."
C. "We can take vitamin A supplements for better effect."
D. "We'll use alcohol-based cleansers for dry skin."

Q268. A child receiving radiation therapy to the head and neck develops difficulty swallowing. Which dietary adjustment is most helpful?

A. Serve soft, bland foods at room temperature
B. Encourage spicy foods to stimulate appetite
C. Provide carbonated beverages between meals
D. Offer dry foods to reduce mucosal irritation

Q269. A child receiving high-dose cytarabine becomes unsteady while walking and has difficulty with coordination. Which nursing action is appropriate?

A. Stop chemotherapy and notify the provider
B. Encourage rest and increase fluids
C. Administer antiemetic therapy
D. Continue therapy and document findings

Q270. A patient receiving anthracycline therapy is prescribed dexrazoxane. What is the purpose of this medication?

A. Enhance chemotherapy efficacy
B. Prevent cardiac toxicity
C. Reduce nausea and vomiting
D. Stimulate white blood cell recovery

Q271. A child undergoing hematopoietic stem cell transplant reports jaundice and weight gain. Which intervention should the nurse implement?

A. Restrict fluids and monitor daily weight
B. Encourage increased fluid intake
C. Administer diuretics as prescribed
D. Provide high-sodium meals

Q272. During administration of rituximab, a child develops fever, chills, and rigors. Which action should the nurse take first?

A. Slow the infusion rate
B. Stop the infusion and assess vital signs
C. Administer corticosteroids
D. Call for emergency support

Q273. A patient receiving cisplatin reports hearing loss. Which diagnostic test should the nurse anticipate?

A. Audiogram
B. Echocardiogram
C. Renal ultrasound
D. Electroencephalogram

Q274. A child develops mild erythema and tenderness at the radiation site. What nursing action is most appropriate?

A. Apply unscented moisturizer to the area
B. Use adhesive tape to secure dressings
C. Clean with alcohol wipes
D. Expose the area to sunlight to promote healing

Q275. A nurse notes a drop in platelet count after chemotherapy. Which action is most appropriate?

A. Provide high-calcium foods
B. Increase physical activity
C. Restrict fluids
D. Institute bleeding precautions

Q276. A child undergoing total body irradiation before transplant reports fatigue and decreased appetite. Which nursing intervention is helpful?

A. Encourage small, nutrient-dense meals and rest periods
B. Increase physical activity
C. Offer carbonated beverages
D. Provide high-fiber foods

Q277. A patient receiving biotherapy for leukemia develops generalized urticaria. What should the nurse do first?

A. Stop the infusion and maintain airway patency
B. Administer antipyretics
C. Continue infusion at half rate
D. Notify the provider after the dose completes

Q278. A nurse caring for a child after stem cell transplant observes dry mouth and thick saliva. What does this indicate?

A. Dehydration
B. Sinusoidal obstruction syndrome
C. Engraftment failure
D. Early mucositis

Q279. A child on methotrexate therapy experiences elevated liver enzymes. Which intervention is appropriate?

A. Notify the provider and hold the next dose
B. Continue the current regimen
C. Encourage high-protein intake
D. Administer mesna prophylactically

Q280. A patient receiving anthracycline chemotherapy reports swelling and redness along the vein after infusion. Which nursing action is most appropriate?

A. Apply cold compresses to the area
B. Elevate the limb and continue infusion
C. Flush the IV line
D. Apply heat to promote absorption

Q281. A child receiving chemotherapy reports mouth pain and white patches on the tongue. Which nursing intervention is most appropriate?

A. Provide alcohol-based mouthwash
B. Encourage citrus beverages
C. Rinse the mouth with saline frequently
D. Offer spicy foods to stimulate appetite

Q282. A child on a morphine infusion for bone pain becomes drowsy and has a respiratory rate of 8 breaths/min. What is the nurse's first action?

A. Stop the infusion and administer naloxone as prescribed
B. Decrease the infusion rate
C. Continue the infusion and reassess in one hour
D. Apply a warm compress to the site

Q283. A patient receiving radiation therapy to the abdomen reports diarrhea and cramping. Which dietary advice is most appropriate?

A. Eat low-residue, low-lactose foods
B. Increase intake of high-fiber vegetables
C. Drink carbonated beverages
D. Consume fried and greasy foods

Q284. A child receiving chemotherapy experiences persistent nausea unrelieved by antiemetics. Which nursing intervention is most effective?

A. Offer the child their favorite food
B. Provide relaxation and distraction techniques
C. Delay all medications
D. Restrict fluids

Q285. A patient undergoing hematopoietic stem cell transplant develops painful urination and hematuria. What should the nurse suspect?

A. Hemorrhagic cystitis
B. Nephrolithiasis
C. Acute glomerulonephritis
D. Urinary tract infection

Q286. A child undergoing treatment for leukemia has a hemoglobin of 6.8 g/dL and

reports fatigue. What is the most appropriate nursing action?

A. Prepare for red blood cell transfusion

B. Encourage increased fluid intake

C. Provide iron-rich foods

D. Encourage deep breathing exercises

Q287. A nurse caring for a child on chemotherapy notes temperature of 38.4°C (101.1°F). What is the nurse's first action?

A. Administer acetaminophen

B. Notify the provider immediately

C. Recheck the temperature in one hour

D. Increase oral fluids

Q288. A patient reports severe fatigue following radiation therapy. Which nursing intervention is most beneficial?

A. Encourage rest periods between activities

B. Promote high-intensity exercise

C. Limit daily fluid intake

D. Encourage large, infrequent meals

Q289. A child receiving chemotherapy complains of tingling in the fingers and toes. What should the nurse do first?

A. Assess safety with ambulation and report symptoms

B. Apply warm compresses

C. Massage extremities to improve circulation

D. Administer acetaminophen

Q290. A nurse is providing education about alopecia related to chemotherapy. Which statement by the parent shows understanding?

A. "Hair loss means treatment is not working."

B. "We will use chemical hair straighteners to reduce hair loss."

C. "We'll cut the hair short after regrowth to prevent shedding."

D. "Hair usually begins to regrow a few months after treatment ends."

Q291. A patient reports constipation while receiving opioid analgesics. Which intervention should the nurse recommend?

A. Encourage a high-fiber diet with adequate fluids

B. Reduce fluid intake to prevent bloating

C. Avoid stool softeners to prevent dependence

D. Limit ambulation to reduce discomfort

Q292. A child receiving vincristine reports difficulty walking and decreased hand grip strength. What should the nurse anticipate?

A. Peripheral neuropathy requiring dose modification

B. Central nervous system relapse

C. Onset of muscle atrophy from inactivity

D. Vascular obstruction

Q293. A patient receiving chemotherapy develops nosebleeds and bruising. Which laboratory finding is expected?

A. Hematocrit of 38%

B. White blood cell count of 8,000/mm^3

C. Platelet count of 20,000/mm^3

D. Sodium level of 138 mEq/L

Q294. A nurse is caring for a patient who reports dyspnea and pallor following chemotherapy. What is the likely cause?

A. Anemia

B. Pulmonary embolism

C. Fluid overload

D. Pneumothorax

Q295. A child undergoing radiation therapy develops pruritus and erythema at the treatment site. What should the nurse recommend?

A. Apply unscented moisturizer and avoid scratching

B. Use talcum powder to keep the area dry

C. Cover the area tightly with dressings

D. Apply alcohol-based lotions

Q296. A patient with sickle cell disease and leukemia reports severe limb pain during vaso-occlusive crisis. What is the most appropriate nursing intervention?

A. Use cold packs for pain relief

B. Restrict fluids

C. Encourage ambulation

D. Administer prescribed opioids and apply heat

Q297. A child receiving chemotherapy has frequent loose stools. Which action should the nurse take?

A. Monitor fluid and electrolyte balance closely

B. Restrict fluid intake

C. Provide high-fiber foods

D. Encourage carbonated drinks

Q298. A patient receiving opioid therapy reports persistent itching. Which intervention is most appropriate?

A. Administer prescribed antihistamines

B. Discontinue opioid therapy

C. Apply cold compresses

D. Reduce fluid intake

Q299. A child receiving chemotherapy presents with cracked lips and bleeding gums. What does this finding indicate?

A. Gingivitis from poor hygiene

B. Vitamin deficiency

C. Oral mucositis

D. Allergic reaction

Q300. A patient undergoing radiation therapy reports decreased appetite and weight loss. Which nursing action is most beneficial?

A. Encourage small, frequent high-calorie meals

B. Offer favorite foods only at mealtime

C. Provide fluids separately from meals

D. Avoid snacks between meals

Answer Key and Explanation (201-300)

Q201. Answer: B

Explanation: Cisplatin can cause ototoxicity due to cochlear hair cell damage, leading to tinnitus and potential hearing loss. Early reporting allows for dose adjustments or discontinuation to prevent irreversible effects. Baseline and periodic audiometric testing are essential in children on platinum-based chemotherapy.

Subdomain: Chemotherapy – Ototoxicity

Q202. Answer: B

Explanation: Interferon causes cytokine-mediated flu-like symptoms such as fever, chills, and malaise. Administering acetaminophen before therapy reduces these effects and improves tolerance. Supportive care includes maintaining hydration and rest between doses.

Subdomain: Biotherapy – Cytokine-Related Effects

Q203. Answer: A

Explanation: Cytokine release syndrome (CRS) is a life-threatening complication of CAR-T therapy caused by a massive immune response. Symptoms include fever, hypotension, and multiorgan dysfunction. Early recognition and treatment with tocilizumab or corticosteroids can prevent progression.

Subdomain: Cellular Therapy – Cytokine Release Syndrome

Q204. Answer: B

Explanation: Neutropenia increases the child's risk of infection, requiring protective precautions. Families should avoid exposure to crowds and individuals with contagious illnesses. Prompt reporting of fever or signs of infection is critical for timely management.

Subdomain: Chemotherapy – Myelosuppression

Q205. Answer: B

Explanation: Radiation-induced somnolence syndrome is a transient post-treatment effect due to delayed demyelination. Symptoms include fatigue, drowsiness, and decreased concentration, resolving spontaneously within weeks. Supportive care with rest and reassurance is typically sufficient.

Subdomain: Radiation Therapy – Neurologic Effects

Q206. Answer: B

Explanation: Doxorubicin is cardiotoxic, potentially leading to decreased left ventricular function and heart failure. Echocardiography is used to monitor ejection fraction before, during, and after therapy. Early detection enables modification of cumulative dosing to prevent irreversible damage.

Subdomain: Chemotherapy – Cardiotoxicity

Q207. Answer: A

Explanation: High-dose cytarabine can cause neurotoxicity due to cerebellar damage, especially in older children or those with renal impairment. Symptoms include ataxia, slurred speech, and altered mental status. Close neurologic monitoring and discontinuation of the drug are essential for recovery.

Subdomain: Chemotherapy – Neurotoxicity

Q208. Answer: B

Explanation: Vincristine is a vesicant, and extravasation can cause severe tissue necrosis. The infusion should be stopped immediately while maintaining IV access for possible antidote administration. The site should be assessed, and institutional extravasation protocols followed promptly.

Subdomain: Chemotherapy – Extravasation Management

Q209. Answer: A

Explanation: Normal saline mouth rinses promote mucosal healing and maintain oral hygiene without irritation. Alcohol and acidic solutions worsen mucosal injury. Pain management and nutritional support are also vital during mucositis recovery.

Subdomain: Hematopoietic Stem Cell Transplantation – Mucosal Toxicity

Q210. Answer: A

Explanation: Etoposide can cause hypotension due to rapid infusion or hypersensitivity reactions. Stopping the infusion and assessing vital signs prevents further hemodynamic compromise. Restarting at a slower rate may be possible after stabilization and provider evaluation.

Subdomain: Chemotherapy – Infusion Reactions

Q211. Answer: A

Explanation: Cyclophosphamide metabolites can irritate the bladder mucosa, leading to hemorrhagic cystitis. Mesna binds toxic metabolites, and adequate hydration promotes renal clearance. Monitoring urine color and ensuring frequent voiding are essential preventive steps.

Subdomain: Chemotherapy – Urologic Toxicity

Q212. Answer: B

Explanation: Gentle cleansing maintains skin integrity and reduces infection risk during radiation dermatitis. Petroleum-based products may worsen irritation by trapping heat. Fragrance-free moisturizers and loose clothing support skin comfort and healing.

Subdomain: Radiation Therapy – Integumentary Effects

Q213. Answer: A

Explanation: Veno-occlusive disease results from hepatic sinusoidal obstruction following conditioning regimens. Clinical signs include hepatomegaly, weight gain, and hyperbilirubinemia. Supportive care with fluid restriction and medications such as defibrotide may be indicated.

Subdomain: Hematopoietic Stem Cell Transplantation – Hepatic Complications

Q214. Answer: A

Explanation: Bleomycin-induced pulmonary toxicity presents as dyspnea and pulmonary infiltrates. Immediate discontinuation and provider notification are required to prevent fibrosis. Baseline and follow-up pulmonary function tests are recommended during therapy.

Subdomain: Chemotherapy – Pulmonary Toxicity

Q215. Answer: C

Explanation: Agents such as vincristine and cisplatin can cause peripheral neuropathy by damaging peripheral nerves. Symptoms include paresthesia and motor weakness. Dose adjustment and safety measures help prevent injury from sensory loss.

Subdomain: Chemotherapy – Neurotoxicity

Q216. Answer: A

Explanation: Urticaria and wheezing indicate a hypersensitivity or anaphylactic reaction. Stopping the infusion and ensuring airway patency are priorities to prevent respiratory collapse. Emergency medications, such as epinephrine and corticosteroids, may be required.

Subdomain: Biotherapy – Hypersensitivity Reactions

Q217. Answer: B

Explanation: Granulocyte colony-stimulating factor (G-CSF) promotes bone marrow recovery by stimulating neutrophil production. It reduces the duration of neutropenia and infection risk following cytotoxic therapy. Bone pain may occur as a side effect due to marrow expansion.

Subdomain: Supportive Therapy – Colony-Stimulating Factors

Q218. Answer: A

Explanation: Intrathecal chemotherapy administration requires dual verification by chemotherapy-certified nurses to prevent fatal errors. Only medications specifically approved for intrathecal use may be administered by this route. Strict adherence to safety protocols ensures patient safety.

Subdomain: Chemotherapy – Safe Handling and Administration

Q219. Answer: A

Explanation: Immunosuppression from chemotherapy predisposes to opportunistic fungal infections like oral candidiasis. Symptoms include white plaques and painful ulcerations. Antifungal therapy and meticulous oral care are key to management.

Subdomain: Chemotherapy – Infectious Complications

Q220. Answer: A

Explanation: Acute graft-versus-host disease (GVHD) occurs when donor T-cells attack host tissues, commonly affecting skin, liver, and gastrointestinal tract. It typically appears within the first 100 days post-transplant. Management includes immunosuppressive therapy and infection prevention measures.

Subdomain: Hematopoietic Stem Cell Transplantation – Graft-Versus-Host Disease

Q221. Answer: C

Explanation: Intrathecal chemotherapy requires independent verification by two chemotherapy-competent nurses to prevent catastrophic

medication errors. This ensures the correct drug, dose, and route are used, as some agents given intrathecally can be fatal. Strict adherence to institutional safety standards is mandatory.
Subdomain: Chemotherapy – Safe Administration Practices

Q222. Answer: B

Explanation: Busulfan can cross the blood-brain barrier and increase the risk of seizures. Prophylactic anticonvulsants are administered to prevent neurologic complications. Early recognition of symptoms allows timely intervention to avoid severe central nervous system toxicity.
Subdomain: Chemotherapy – Neurotoxicity

Q223. Answer: B

Explanation: Acute graft-versus-host disease results from donor lymphocytes attacking host tissues, particularly the skin, liver, and gastrointestinal tract. The combination of rash and profuse diarrhea is characteristic. Prompt recognition and immunosuppressive therapy are essential to prevent severe organ involvement.
Subdomain: Hematopoietic Stem Cell Transplantation – Acute GVHD

Q224. Answer: A

Explanation: Bleomycin may cause pulmonary fibrosis, particularly at high cumulative doses. Pulmonary function testing and chest imaging help assess lung toxicity. Early identification of respiratory changes allows discontinuation of the drug to minimize long-term damage.
Subdomain: Chemotherapy – Pulmonary Toxicity

Q225. Answer: C

Explanation: Dyspnea on exertion may indicate reduced left ventricular function secondary to anthracycline-induced cardiomyopathy. Baseline and ongoing echocardiograms are used to detect early cardiac changes. Dose limitation and dexrazoxane may reduce long-term cardiac injury risk.
Subdomain: Chemotherapy – Cardiotoxicity

Q226. Answer: B

Explanation: Vincristine commonly causes peripheral neuropathy manifested by motor weakness and loss of reflexes. Early reporting allows dose modification to prevent permanent deficits. Supportive care includes fall prevention and physical therapy as needed.
Subdomain: Chemotherapy – Neurotoxicity

Q227. Answer: A

Explanation: Cytarabine can cause chemical conjunctivitis due to direct irritation of the ocular mucosa. Prophylactic or therapeutic corticosteroid eye drops minimize inflammation and discomfort. Eye care is essential when administering high-dose cytarabine regimens.
Subdomain: Chemotherapy – Ocular Toxicity

Q228. Answer: B

Explanation: Prophylactic antiemetic administration before radiation helps prevent nausea and vomiting related to gastrointestinal mucosal irritation. Consistent scheduling of antiemetics optimizes symptom control. Encouraging hydration supports tolerance to treatment.
Subdomain: Radiation Therapy – Gastrointestinal Side Effects

Q229. Answer: A

Explanation: Fever and chills during monoclonal antibody infusion indicate an infusion-related reaction caused by cytokine release. The infusion should be stopped and vital signs assessed. Premedication with antipyretics and antihistamines can prevent recurrence.
Subdomain: Biotherapy – Infusion Reactions

Q230. Answer: C

Explanation: Leucovorin acts as a folinic acid rescue to replenish folate stores depleted by methotrexate, protecting normal tissues from toxic effects. Timely administration is crucial to avoid myelosuppression and mucositis. Serum methotrexate levels guide the duration of rescue therapy.
Subdomain: Chemotherapy – Toxicity Management

Q231. Answer: B

Explanation: Thrombocytopenia is a common side effect of chemotherapy that leads to easy bruising and bleeding. Monitoring platelet counts helps guide transfusion needs and activity restrictions. Safety education for the family focuses on preventing injury and bleeding episodes.
Subdomain: Chemotherapy – Myelosuppression

Q232. Answer: C

Explanation: Hematuria and dysuria during chemotherapy may indicate hemorrhagic cystitis, often associated with cyclophosphamide or ifosfamide. Prompt provider notification allows initiation of diagnostic and protective interventions, such as mesna administration and hydration. Early action prevents severe bladder damage.

Subdomain: Chemotherapy – Urologic Toxicity

Q233. Answer: A

Explanation: Engraftment syndrome occurs during marrow recovery and is characterized by fever, rash, and pulmonary edema due to cytokine release. Supportive care with corticosteroids is often required. Differentiating this from infection is crucial for appropriate treatment.

Subdomain: Hematopoietic Stem Cell Transplantation – Engraftment Syndrome

Q234. Answer: D

Explanation: Vincristine disrupts microtubule formation, leading to peripheral neuropathy. Symptoms include paresthesias, weakness, and motor impairment. Monitoring neurologic function and adjusting dosage can prevent long-term disability.

Subdomain: Chemotherapy – Peripheral Neuropathy

Q235. Answer: A

Explanation: Hypotension during biotherapy infusion suggests an acute hypersensitivity or cytokine-mediated reaction. The infusion must be stopped immediately, and vital signs closely monitored. Supportive management includes oxygen, fluids, and possible administration of corticosteroids or epinephrine.

Subdomain: Biotherapy – Hypersensitivity Reaction

Q236. Answer: B

Explanation: A low-lactose, low-residue diet minimizes bowel stimulation and helps control radiation-induced diarrhea. Patients should avoid high-fiber foods and maintain hydration. Small, frequent meals improve tolerance and comfort.

Subdomain: Radiation Therapy – Gastrointestinal Effects

Q237. Answer: A

Explanation: Graft-versus-host disease occurs when donor T-cells attack host tissues, often presenting with skin rash and liver dysfunction. Early detection allows immunosuppressive therapy to reduce severity. Monitoring liver enzymes and skin integrity is essential.

Subdomain: Hematopoietic Stem Cell Transplantation – GVHD

Q238. Answer: A

Explanation: Erythema and swelling at the infusion site may indicate extravasation, especially with vesicant agents. Immediate cessation of infusion and assessment of the site prevent tissue necrosis. Institutional protocols should be followed for antidote administration and care.

Subdomain: Chemotherapy – Extravasation Management

Q239. Answer: D

Explanation: Cyclophosphamide metabolites irritate the bladder, increasing risk for hemorrhagic cystitis. Encouraging frequent voiding and hydration helps flush toxins from the urinary tract. Families should report any hematuria or dysuria immediately.

Subdomain: Chemotherapy – Urologic Toxicity Prevention

Q240. Answer: A

Explanation: These findings suggest sinusoidal obstruction syndrome, a hepatic complication after transplantation. Fluid restriction and daily weight monitoring help manage hepatic congestion. Early intervention reduces risk of progressive liver failure.

Subdomain: Hematopoietic Stem Cell Transplantation – Hepatic Complications

Q241. Answer: B

Explanation: Hematuria may indicate hemorrhagic cystitis caused by toxic metabolites of ifosfamide. Immediate provider notification allows for rapid initiation of mesna and hydration to prevent bladder damage. Early intervention is critical to avoid long-term urinary complications.

Subdomain: Chemotherapy – Urologic Toxicity

Q242. Answer: C

Explanation: Cisplatin often causes severe, prolonged nausea and vomiting that may require combination antiemetic therapy targeting different pathways. Using both serotonin receptor antagonists and neurokinin-1 inhibitors improves symptom control. Adequate hydration supports treatment tolerance.
Subdomain: Chemotherapy – Gastrointestinal Effects

Q243. Answer: C

Explanation: CAR-T cell therapy may lead to immune effector cell-associated neurotoxicity (ICANS), characterized by confusion, aphasia, and seizures. The pathophysiology involves cytokine-mediated brain inflammation. Early neurologic assessment and supportive management are essential to prevent severe complications.
Subdomain: Cellular Therapy – Neurotoxicity

Q244. Answer: A

Explanation: Radiation-induced xerosis and desquamation require gentle skin care with nonirritating, fragrance-free emollients. Alcohol-based products should be avoided as they dry and irritate the skin. Patient education focuses on protecting the irradiated area from trauma and sun exposure.
Subdomain: Radiation Therapy – Integumentary Effects

Q245. Answer: B

Explanation: Doxorubicin can cause dose-related cardiotoxicity by damaging myocardial cells. Routine cardiac monitoring ensures early detection of decreased ejection fraction or heart failure. Adjusting dosage or using cardioprotective agents can prevent irreversible damage.
Subdomain: Chemotherapy – Cardiotoxicity

Q246. Answer: B

Explanation: Fever in an immunocompromised patient may indicate infection and requires prompt evaluation and empiric antibiotics. Although bone pain is expected with G-CSF, fever is an emergency. Early management prevents sepsis in neutropenic patients.
Subdomain: Supportive Therapy – Infection Risk Management

Q247. Answer: D

Explanation: Elevated creatinine indicates renal toxicity leading to delayed methotrexate clearance. Increasing leucovorin rescue protects healthy cells from toxic effects. Aggressive hydration and urine alkalinization are also essential for renal recovery.
Subdomain: Chemotherapy – Nephrotoxicity

Q248. Answer: B

Explanation: Biotherapy-related cytokine release often causes fever, chills, and rigors. Antihistamines such as diphenhydramine help reduce symptoms and prevent escalation to severe reactions. Pre-infusion medications are often used prophylactically in high-risk patients.
Subdomain: Biotherapy – Infusion Reactions

Q249. Answer: A

Explanation: High-dose cytarabine can cause cerebellar toxicity, resulting in ataxia and speech disturbances. Immediate cessation of therapy and neurologic evaluation are necessary to prevent irreversible injury. Regular neuro checks during therapy are standard practice.
Subdomain: Chemotherapy – Neurotoxicity

Q250. Answer: A

Explanation: Etoposide may cause hypotension when infused too rapidly. Stopping the infusion and monitoring the patient's hemodynamic status prevents cardiovascular compromise. Restarting at a slower rate after stabilization is usually safe.
Subdomain: Chemotherapy – Infusion Reactions

Q251. Answer: D

Explanation: Adequate hydration is vital to prevent bladder irritation from cyclophosphamide metabolites. Encouraging frequent voiding reduces the risk of hemorrhagic cystitis. Families should report hematuria promptly to healthcare providers.
Subdomain: Chemotherapy – Urologic Toxicity Prevention

Q252. Answer: A

Explanation: Isotretinoin causes mucocutaneous dryness, including chapped lips and dry skin, due to its retinoid effects. Monitoring hydration and providing moisturizers help relieve discomfort. Patients should also avoid vitamin A supplements to prevent toxicity.

Subdomain: Maintenance Therapy – Retinoid Side Effects

Q253. Answer: B

Explanation: Sinusoidal obstruction syndrome presents with hepatomegaly, ascites, and hyperbilirubinemia after high-dose conditioning regimens. The condition results from hepatic venule injury and impaired venous outflow. Supportive management includes fluid restriction and defibrotide.

Subdomain: Hematopoietic Stem Cell Transplantation – Hepatic Complications

Q254. Answer: A

Explanation: Radiation-induced mucositis requires a soft, bland diet and frequent saline rinses to minimize irritation. Acidic or spicy foods worsen pain and tissue breakdown. Maintaining oral hygiene supports healing and infection prevention.

Subdomain: Radiation Therapy – Oral Mucositis

Q255. Answer: A

Explanation: Redness and swelling suggest possible extravasation, especially with vesicant drugs. Stopping the infusion immediately prevents further tissue damage. Institutional extravasation management protocols should be followed.

Subdomain: Chemotherapy – Extravasation Management

Q256. Answer: D

Explanation: Hematuria is a hallmark sign of hemorrhagic cystitis from cyclophosphamide metabolites. Monitoring urine for blood allows early detection and treatment. Preventive measures include hydration and administration of mesna.

Subdomain: Chemotherapy – Urologic Complications

Q257. Answer: A

Explanation: Trimethoprim-sulfamethoxazole delays methotrexate clearance, increasing the risk of toxicity. Avoiding this combination prevents severe myelosuppression and mucositis. Careful medication reconciliation is essential during chemotherapy.

Subdomain: Chemotherapy – Drug Interactions

Q258. Answer: A

Explanation: Fatigue and mood changes are common biotherapy side effects caused by cytokine release. Supportive interventions include rest, psychosocial support, and reassurance. Education about symptom expectations promotes adherence to treatment.

Subdomain: Biotherapy – Psychosocial Effects

Q259. Answer: C

Explanation: Fever is often the earliest and most important sign of infection in immunocompromised patients. Immediate evaluation and initiation of antibiotics are critical to prevent sepsis. Routine temperature monitoring is essential during neutropenia.

Subdomain: Hematopoietic Stem Cell Transplantation – Infection Management

Q260. Answer: A

Explanation: Anticipatory nausea arises from conditioned anxiety responses related to prior treatment experiences. Combining antiemetics with behavioral strategies like relaxation and guided imagery helps minimize symptoms. Psychological support enhances tolerance of future treatments.

Subdomain: Radiation Therapy – Anticipatory Nausea Management

Q261. Answer: C

Explanation: Ifosfamide can cause neurotoxicity due to its metabolite, chloroacetaldehyde, leading to encephalopathy. Symptoms include confusion, somnolence, and hallucinations. Stopping the drug and administering methylene blue may reverse symptoms.

Subdomain: Chemotherapy – Neurotoxicity

Q262. Answer: B

Explanation: Stomatitis and mucositis are common methotrexate toxicities due to folate depletion in rapidly dividing cells. Increasing leucovorin rescue helps mitigate toxicity and promote mucosal healing. Oral care and pain management are also key supportive measures.

Subdomain: Chemotherapy – Mucosal Toxicity

Q263. Answer: B

Explanation: Acute graft-versus-host disease typically occurs within the first 100 days post-transplant and affects the skin, gastrointestinal tract, and liver. Early symptoms include rash,

diarrhea, and jaundice. Prompt immunosuppressive therapy reduces morbidity.
Subdomain: Hematopoietic Stem Cell Transplantation – GVHD

Q264. Answer: A

Explanation: Bleomycin toxicity damages lung tissue, leading to interstitial pneumonitis and fibrosis. Pulmonary function tests and imaging evaluate the extent of injury. Monitoring during therapy helps identify toxicity early, allowing treatment modification.
Subdomain: Chemotherapy – Pulmonary Toxicity

Q265. Answer: A

Explanation: Mesna binds acrolein, the urotoxic metabolite of cyclophosphamide, preventing bladder irritation and hemorrhagic cystitis. It must be administered with or shortly after chemotherapy. Hydration and frequent voiding further protect bladder integrity.
Subdomain: Chemotherapy – Urologic Toxicity Prevention

Q266. Answer: B

Explanation: Doxorubicin is a vesicant, and extravasation can cause severe tissue necrosis. The infusion should be stopped immediately, and the site assessed for damage. Cold compresses and antidotes such as dexrazoxane may be required.
Subdomain: Chemotherapy – Extravasation Management

Q267. Answer: A

Explanation: Retinoids increase skin sensitivity and dryness, making sun protection essential. Patients should use sunscreen, avoid harsh cleansers, and maintain hydration. Vitamin A supplements should be avoided to prevent toxicity.
Subdomain: Maintenance Therapy – Retinoid Toxicity

Q268. Answer: A

Explanation: Oropharyngeal mucositis from radiation causes pain and dysphagia. Soft, bland foods reduce irritation and promote nutritional intake. Avoiding spicy or acidic foods minimizes discomfort during swallowing.
Subdomain: Radiation Therapy – Oral Toxicity

Q269. Answer: A

Explanation: Cerebellar toxicity from high-dose cytarabine manifests as ataxia and coordination problems. The drug should be stopped immediately, and neurologic evaluation obtained. Frequent neuro assessments are required during therapy.
Subdomain: Chemotherapy – Neurotoxicity

Q270. Answer: B

Explanation: Dexrazoxane acts as a cardioprotective agent by chelating free radicals formed by anthracycline metabolism. It reduces the risk of cardiomyopathy without interfering with antitumor effects. Routine cardiac monitoring remains essential.
Subdomain: Chemotherapy – Cardiotoxicity Prevention

Q271. Answer: A

Explanation: These symptoms suggest sinusoidal obstruction syndrome due to hepatic venous congestion. Fluid restriction and close monitoring help manage volume overload. Early intervention prevents progression to liver failure.
Subdomain: Hematopoietic Stem Cell Transplantation – Hepatic Complications

Q272. Answer: B

Explanation: Rituximab can cause infusion-related reactions, including fever and chills due to cytokine release. Stopping the infusion allows assessment and stabilization of the patient. Restarting at a slower rate after symptom resolution is often appropriate.
Subdomain: Biotherapy – Infusion Reaction

Q273. Answer: A

Explanation: Cisplatin can cause ototoxicity by damaging cochlear hair cells, leading to tinnitus and hearing loss. Baseline and serial audiograms monitor auditory function. Early detection supports dose modification to prevent permanent loss.
Subdomain: Chemotherapy – Ototoxicity

Q274. Answer: A

Explanation: Radiation dermatitis is best managed with gentle skin care and fragrance-free moisturizers. Patients should avoid harsh chemicals, friction, and direct sunlight. Education helps prevent worsening of skin reactions.

Subdomain: Radiation Therapy – Skin Integrity Management

Q275. Answer: D

Explanation: Thrombocytopenia increases bleeding risk during chemotherapy. Implementing bleeding precautions, such as using soft toothbrushes and avoiding invasive procedures, minimizes complications. Monitoring platelet counts guides transfusion decisions.

Subdomain: Chemotherapy – Myelosuppression

Q276. Answer: A

Explanation: Fatigue and anorexia are common side effects of radiation. Encouraging rest and small, frequent meals supports energy and nutrition. Balanced care promotes tolerance and recovery.

Subdomain: Radiation Therapy – Fatigue Management

Q277. Answer: A

Explanation: Urticaria indicates a hypersensitivity or anaphylactic reaction to biotherapy. Immediate cessation of infusion and airway management are priorities. Emergency medications such as epinephrine and corticosteroids may be required.

Subdomain: Biotherapy – Hypersensitivity Reactions

Q278. Answer: D

Explanation: Mucositis from chemotherapy or radiation often begins with dryness and thickened oral secretions. Early identification allows preventive measures like saline rinses and oral hygiene. Pain control and infection prevention are key to care.

Subdomain: Hematopoietic Stem Cell Transplantation – Mucosal Toxicity

Q279. Answer: A

Explanation: Methotrexate can cause hepatotoxicity, indicated by elevated transaminases. Holding the medication and notifying the provider prevent progression to hepatic injury. Regular monitoring ensures safe continuation of therapy.

Subdomain: Chemotherapy – Hepatotoxicity

Q280. Answer: A

Explanation: Redness and swelling following anthracycline infusion indicate possible extravasation. Cold compresses help limit tissue injury by reducing drug spread. The provider should be notified for evaluation and potential antidote use.

Subdomain: Chemotherapy – Extravasation Management

Q281. Answer: C

Explanation: Chemotherapy can cause mucositis and opportunistic infections such as oral candidiasis. Frequent saline rinses maintain oral hygiene and reduce discomfort without irritating the mucosa. Acidic and alcohol-based products worsen inflammation and should be avoided.

Subdomain: Oral Mucositis Management

Q282. Answer: A

Explanation: Opioid toxicity causes sedation and respiratory depression, requiring immediate discontinuation and reversal with naloxone. Close monitoring and reassessment are essential to prevent respiratory arrest. Supportive oxygen therapy may be required during recovery.

Subdomain: Pain Management – Opioid Safety

Q283. Answer: A

Explanation: Radiation to the gastrointestinal tract causes mucosal inflammation, resulting in diarrhea and malabsorption. A low-residue, low-lactose diet reduces bowel stimulation and improves tolerance. Adequate hydration and small, frequent meals are also recommended.

Subdomain: Gastrointestinal Symptom Management

Q284. Answer: B

Explanation: Nonpharmacologic interventions such as relaxation, guided imagery, and distraction complement antiemetic therapy and help manage anticipatory or refractory nausea. Reducing anxiety can lessen the severity of symptoms. Maintaining hydration prevents further complications.

Subdomain: Nausea and Vomiting – Supportive Measures

Q285. Answer: A

Explanation: Hemorrhagic cystitis is a known complication of cyclophosphamide, ifosfamide, and viral reactivation after transplant. It presents with dysuria, hematuria, and suprapubic pain. Prevention includes hydration, mesna, and antiviral prophylaxis.

Subdomain: Urologic Symptom Management

Q286. Answer: A

Explanation: Severe anemia from chemotherapy-induced bone marrow suppression requires red blood cell transfusion to restore oxygen-carrying capacity. Monitoring for transfusion reactions and evaluating post-transfusion response are key nursing responsibilities.

Subdomain: Hematologic Supportive Care

Q287. Answer: B

Explanation: Fever in a neutropenic patient is a medical emergency indicating potential sepsis. Immediate provider notification and initiation of broad-spectrum antibiotics are critical to prevent rapid deterioration. Antipyretics should be avoided until cultures are obtained.

Subdomain: Infection Management – Febrile Neutropenia

Q288. Answer: A

Explanation: Fatigue is a common treatment-related symptom resulting from metabolic changes and tissue repair demands. Encouraging rest and balancing activity promote energy conservation. Nutritional support and emotional encouragement enhance recovery.

Subdomain: Fatigue Management

Q289. Answer: A

Explanation: Peripheral neuropathy from neurotoxic agents such as vincristine requires safety assessment and provider notification for possible dose adjustment. Early recognition prevents injury and functional decline. Physical therapy may help maintain strength and coordination.

Subdomain: Neuropathy Management

Q290. Answer: D

Explanation: Chemotherapy-induced alopecia is temporary, and hair typically begins to regrow within 2–3 months after therapy completion. Providing anticipatory guidance and emotional support helps children and families cope with the visible side effects.

Subdomain: Body Image and Coping Support

Q291. Answer: A

Explanation: Opioid-induced constipation results from slowed gastrointestinal motility. A high-fiber diet, increased fluids, and stool softeners prevent discomfort and fecal impaction. Physical activity also supports bowel regularity.

Subdomain: Gastrointestinal Symptom Management

Q292. Answer: A

Explanation: Vincristine can cause dose-related peripheral neuropathy, leading to motor weakness and sensory deficits. Early recognition allows for dose adjustments to prevent permanent impairment. Safety precautions and supportive therapy improve function.

Subdomain: Neuropathy and Motor Function Support

Q293. Answer: C

Explanation: Thrombocytopenia is a common adverse effect of chemotherapy, leading to increased bleeding risk. Monitoring platelet counts and implementing bleeding precautions are essential nursing measures. Platelet transfusions may be required for severe cases.

Subdomain: Hematologic Supportive Care

Q294. Answer: A

Explanation: Chemotherapy-induced anemia results from bone marrow suppression, reducing oxygen delivery to tissues. Symptoms include fatigue, pallor, and dyspnea. Transfusion and energy conservation strategies improve oxygenation.

Subdomain: Fatigue and Anemia Management

Q295. Answer: A

Explanation: Radiation dermatitis requires gentle care with nonirritating moisturizers to maintain skin integrity. Scratching and tight coverings exacerbate irritation and delay healing. Patients should avoid sun exposure and harsh products.

Subdomain: Integumentary Symptom Management

Q296. Answer: D

Explanation: Vaso-occlusive pain results from ischemia due to sickled cells obstructing blood flow. Opioid analgesics and heat therapy relieve pain and promote vasodilation. Adequate hydration helps prevent recurrence of crisis episodes.

Subdomain: Pain and Crisis Management

Q297. Answer: A

Explanation: Chemotherapy-induced diarrhea increases risk for dehydration and electrolyte imbalances. Strict monitoring and appropriate fluid replacement are critical. A bland, low-fiber diet helps reduce stool frequency.
Subdomain: Fluid and Electrolyte Balance

Q298. Answer: A

Explanation: Pruritus is a common opioid side effect caused by histamine release. Antihistamines provide effective symptomatic relief without altering analgesic benefits. Monitoring for sedation and respiratory depression remains important.
Subdomain: Pain Management – Side Effect Control

Q299. Answer: C

Explanation: Oral mucositis results from chemotherapy-induced injury to the mucosal lining, causing ulcerations and bleeding. Regular saline rinses, pain control, and avoidance of irritants promote healing. Preventive oral care reduces infection risk.
Subdomain: Oral and Mucosal Care

Q300. Answer: A

Explanation: Anorexia and early satiety are common during radiation therapy. Encouraging small, nutrient-dense meals throughout the day supports caloric intake. Collaboration with a dietitian ensures optimal nutritional management.
Subdomain: Nutritional Support and Appetite Management

Question (301-400)

Q301. A child receiving chemotherapy reports a metallic taste and loss of appetite. Which intervention is most helpful?

A. Offer cold foods and use plastic utensils
B. Serve meals with strong seasonings
C. Encourage high-fat meals
D. Provide citrus beverages before meals

Q302. A child receiving morphine for postoperative pain becomes confused and agitated. What is the nurse's priority action?

A. Administer naloxone immediately
B. Continue the infusion as prescribed
C. Offer reassurance and reorientation
D. Assess for hypoxia and respiratory status

Q303. A patient with leukemia reports mild anxiety before chemotherapy sessions. Which nursing intervention is most effective?

A. Use guided imagery and deep breathing exercises
B. Limit family visits before treatment
C. Administer sedatives prophylactically
D. Encourage avoidance of treatment discussions

Q304. A child undergoing radiation therapy develops dry mouth and thick saliva. What nursing action is appropriate?

A. Encourage frequent sips of water and sugar-free gum
B. Offer salted snacks to stimulate saliva
C. Restrict oral intake
D. Provide mouth rinses containing alcohol

Q305. A child receiving vincristine reports constipation and abdominal discomfort. What should the nurse recommend?

A. Limit activity until symptoms resolve
B. Increase fiber and fluid intake
C. Reduce fluid intake to prevent bloating
D. Administer opioids for pain relief

Q306. A nurse notes that a child receiving chemotherapy has developed a nosebleed. Which intervention should the nurse implement first?

A. Apply firm pressure to the bridge of the nose
B. Insert cotton swabs into the nostrils
C. Tilt the head backward
D. Pack the nose with petroleum gauze

Q307. A patient undergoing chemotherapy complains of numbness in fingertips and difficulty with buttons. Which safety teaching is most appropriate?

A. Use nonslip footwear and assistive devices
B. Avoid all physical activity
C. Increase hand exercises and use heat
D. Report symptoms only if severe

Q308. A child on long-term corticosteroid therapy develops facial rounding and weight gain. Which nursing intervention is indicated?

A. Discontinue corticosteroids immediately
B. Reduce caloric intake drastically
C. Encourage strenuous exercise
D. Provide nutritional counseling and monitor glucose levels

Q309. A child receiving cranial radiation complains of headache and fatigue several weeks after treatment. What condition should the nurse suspect?

A. Somnolence syndrome
B. Tumor recurrence
C. Intracranial hemorrhage
D. Medication withdrawal

Q310. A patient undergoing chemotherapy reports decreased concentration and memory difficulties. What supportive strategy is best?

A. Use planners and written reminders for tasks
B. Encourage complete bed rest
C. Increase caffeine intake
D. Avoid mental activities to prevent fatigue

Q311. A child with a mediport reports tenderness and redness around the site. What is the priority nursing action?

A. Apply warm compresses
B. Flush the line to clear obstruction
C. Assess for infection and obtain cultures
D. Administer scheduled chemotherapy

Q312. A child with sickle cell disease and leukemia reports severe bone pain. Which collaborative intervention provides the most effective relief?

A. Administer opioid analgesics and apply heat
B. Restrict fluids and use cold packs
C. Encourage vigorous activity
D. Apply ice and elevation to the area

Q313. A patient receiving chemotherapy reports ringing in the ears. Which agent is most likely responsible?
A. Cisplatin
B. Doxorubicin
C. Methotrexate
D. Etoposide
Q314. A patient undergoing hematopoietic stem cell transplant develops a rash and diarrhea during engraftment. What should the nurse suspect?
A. Viral exanthem
B. Graft-versus-host disease
C. Sinusoidal obstruction syndrome
D. Allergic drug reaction
Q315. A child receiving opioid therapy reports new-onset itching. Which intervention is appropriate?
A. Administer antihistamines as prescribed
B. Discontinue the opioid immediately
C. Reduce oral fluid intake
D. Apply ice to the affected area
Q316. A patient receiving chemotherapy develops hand-foot syndrome with redness and peeling on palms and soles. What should the nurse recommend?
A. Avoid heat and friction on affected areas
B. Use alcohol-based lotions twice daily
C. Increase physical activity
D. Apply ice directly to the skin
Q317. A nurse notes shallow breathing and pinpoint pupils in a child receiving morphine. What is the nurse's immediate action?
A. Notify provider without intervening
B. Continue morphine and monitor
C. Provide deep breathing exercises
D. Administer naloxone per protocol
Q318. A patient reports difficulty sleeping during chemotherapy. Which nonpharmacologic intervention is most effective?
A. Maintain a consistent bedtime routine
B. Increase caffeine intake to reduce fatigue
C. Watch television in bed until drowsy
D. Sleep during the day to catch up on rest
Q319. A child receiving radiation therapy complains of painful swallowing. What nursing intervention is indicated?
A. Provide soft, bland foods and saline rinses
B. Encourage acidic fruit juices
C. Offer hard crackers to promote saliva
D. Limit oral intake to reduce pain
Q320. A child with neutropenia after chemotherapy develops mouth ulcers. What dietary advice should the nurse provide?
A. Drink unpasteurized juices for vitamins
B. Eat high-fiber foods for healing
C. Avoid raw fruits and vegetables
D. Include rare-cooked meats for protein
Q321. A child receiving chemotherapy complains of tingling and burning in the feet. What should the nurse do first?
A. Apply warm compresses to the extremities
B. Assess gait and balance during ambulation
C. Administer antiemetics as prescribed
D. Encourage increased fluid intake
Q322. A patient receiving radiation therapy develops painful skin lesions within the treatment field. Which intervention should the nurse implement?
A. Apply nonadherent dressings to affected areas
B. Clean the skin with alcohol wipes
C. Apply heat packs to the lesions
D. Cover the area tightly with bandages
Q323. A child receiving methotrexate develops stomatitis and oral ulcers. Which nursing action is most appropriate?
A. Encourage saline mouth rinses several times daily
B. Provide lemon-flavored mouthwash
C. Increase intake of spicy foods
D. Use hydrogen peroxide rinses
Q324. A child undergoing hematopoietic stem cell transplant develops a sudden temperature of 38.5°C (101.3°F). What should the nurse do immediately?
A. Encourage oral fluids
B. Administer acetaminophen for fever
C. Notify the provider and obtain blood cultures
D. Recheck temperature after 1 hour
Q325. A child receiving doxorubicin reports shortness of breath and fatigue. What is the nurse's best action?
A. Notify the provider for cardiac evaluation
B. Encourage deep breathing exercises

C. Provide supplemental oxygen and continue therapy
D. Reassure that symptoms are temporary

Q326. A nurse is teaching a parent how to manage a child's nausea during chemotherapy. Which instruction is most appropriate?
A. Offer small, frequent meals of bland foods
B. Encourage spicy and greasy foods for calories
C. Restrict all fluid intake before therapy
D. Avoid antiemetics unless nausea is severe

Q327. A child undergoing radiation therapy reports extreme tiredness. Which nursing recommendation is best?
A. Restrict fluids to minimize swelling
B. Encourage high-intensity exercise
C. Discourage naps during the day
D. Alternate activity with rest periods throughout the day

Q328. A nurse caring for a child with mucositis notes bleeding gums and petechiae. Which laboratory result should be reviewed first?
A. Platelet count
B. Hemoglobin level
C. Sodium level
D. Glucose level

Q329. A patient receiving cisplatin reports persistent ringing in the ears. Which nursing action is appropriate?
A. Report findings and schedule audiometric evaluation
B. Administer pain medication
C. Encourage increased hydration
D. Reassure that symptoms will resolve spontaneously

Q330. A child receiving opioids for cancer pain reports constipation despite stool softeners. What should the nurse recommend next?
A. Encourage rest and minimal movement
B. Discontinue opioid therapy
C. Limit fluid intake
D. Add a stimulant laxative to the regimen

Q331. A patient with leukemia reports sudden shortness of breath after transfusion. What complication should the nurse suspect?
A. Transfusion-related acute lung injury (TRALI)
B. Hypervolemia
C. Bacterial pneumonia
D. Pulmonary embolism

Q332. A nurse caring for a neutropenic patient observes a temperature of 38°C (100.4°F). What is the most critical next step?
A. Obtain blood cultures and start antibiotics promptly
B. Provide warm blankets and recheck later
C. Administer acetaminophen and fluids
D. Encourage the patient to ambulate

Q333. A patient undergoing chemotherapy reports frequent urination and intense thirst. Which laboratory value should the nurse monitor?
A. Serum calcium
B. Hemoglobin
C. Blood glucose
D. Platelet count

Q334. A child with mucositis refuses to eat due to mouth pain. Which intervention supports nutritional intake?
A. Provide cool, bland foods and oral rinses before meals
B. Offer hot, spicy foods to stimulate appetite
C. Encourage citrus juices to aid healing
D. Withhold all oral intake until pain resolves

Q335. A patient receiving total parenteral nutrition develops shortness of breath and chest pain. What should the nurse do first?
A. Stop the infusion and place the patient in left lateral Trendelenburg position
B. Recheck infusion rate
C. Administer oxygen and continue therapy
D. Flush the catheter aggressively

Q336. A child receiving chemotherapy has mouth ulcers and neutropenia. Which dietary precaution is necessary?
A. Offer homemade yogurt for probiotics
B. Provide fresh salads to improve nutrition
C. Encourage rare-cooked meats
D. Avoid raw fruits, vegetables, and unpasteurized foods

Q337. A child receiving methotrexate therapy complains of severe fatigue. What is the nurse's best intervention?
A. Evaluate hemoglobin levels and assess for anemia
B. Encourage high-intensity physical activity
C. Administer stimulant medication
D. Restrict daytime naps

Q338. A patient undergoing chemotherapy complains of numbness and difficulty writing. Which teaching should the nurse provide?

A. Use adaptive utensils and avoid tasks requiring fine motor skills

B. Increase physical exertion to restore circulation

C. Apply heat compresses for relief

D. Ignore mild symptoms unless severe

Q339. A patient receiving radiation therapy reports dry, itchy scalp and hair loss. What should the nurse advise?

A. Wash scalp daily with hot water

B. Use gentle, fragrance-free shampoo and protect scalp from sun

C. Apply alcohol-based hair tonic

D. Use tight head coverings

Q340. A child receiving chemotherapy presents with dark-colored urine and flank pain. What complication should the nurse suspect?

A. Tumor lysis syndrome

B. Urinary tract infection

C. Hepatic failure

D. Dehydration

Q341. A child receiving cyclophosphamide reports pain with urination and blood in the urine. What nursing action is most appropriate?

A. Increase hydration and report findings immediately

B. Apply warm compresses to the abdomen

C. Encourage the child to delay urination

D. Restrict fluids for comfort

Q342. A nurse observes that a child undergoing total body irradiation has a poor appetite and weight loss. Which nursing intervention is most effective?

A. Provide large meals three times per day

B. Offer food only when the child is hungry

C. Restrict fluids during meals

D. Encourage small, frequent, high-calorie meals

Q343. A patient undergoing chemotherapy reports frequent nosebleeds. Which laboratory result should the nurse review first?

A. Platelet count

B. White blood cell count

C. Serum sodium

D. Hemoglobin level

Q344. A child receiving opioid analgesia for cancer pain develops nausea and vomiting. Which intervention should the nurse implement?

A. Administer prescribed antiemetic and reassess effectiveness

B. Discontinue opioid therapy

C. Reduce oral fluid intake

D. Encourage the child to lie flat after dosing

Q345. A patient undergoing radiation therapy to the abdomen reports persistent diarrhea. What dietary recommendation is most appropriate?

A. Drink carbonated beverages frequently

B. Increase intake of raw vegetables and fruits

C. Consume a low-fiber, lactose-free diet

D. Avoid all dairy products permanently

Q346. A nurse is caring for a child receiving methotrexate who reports fatigue and pallor. Which assessment finding should the nurse anticipate?

A. Low hemoglobin and hematocrit

B. Elevated white blood cell count

C. High platelet count

D. Increased urine output

Q347. A patient undergoing chemotherapy develops oral ulcers and difficulty eating. Which intervention should the nurse prioritize?

A. Provide topical anesthetics before meals

B. Offer hot soups and spicy foods

C. Use alcohol-based rinses twice daily

D. Restrict all oral intake until healed

Q348. A child receiving high-dose cytarabine experiences confusion and slurred speech. What should the nurse do first?

A. Provide reassurance and monitor

B. Administer antiemetics

C. Encourage oral fluids

D. Stop the chemotherapy and notify the provider

Q349. A nurse is caring for a patient on biotherapy who develops chills, fever, and rigors during infusion. What is the first nursing action?

A. Stop the infusion and assess vital signs

B. Continue infusion at half the rate

C. Administer corticosteroids immediately

D. Increase IV fluids

Q350. A child receiving vincristine reports constipation for three days. Which medication should the nurse anticipate administering?
A. A stool softener and mild stimulant laxative
B. An opioid analgesic
C. Antihistamine
D. Proton pump inhibitor

Q351. A patient with sickle cell disease develops chest pain, cough, and fever. What complication should the nurse suspect?
A. Pulmonary embolism
B. Acute chest syndrome
C. Pneumothorax
D. Bronchitis

Q352. A child receiving chemotherapy presents with severe bone pain after filgrastim administration. Which action is most appropriate?
A. Administer acetaminophen as prescribed
B. Stop filgrastim immediately
C. Apply cold compresses
D. Encourage weight-bearing exercise

Q353. A nurse caring for a child with nausea and vomiting after chemotherapy wants to prevent anticipatory symptoms. Which strategy is most effective?
A. Administer antiemetics before each chemotherapy session
B. Restrict oral intake the night before treatment
C. Limit discussions about treatment
D. Offer antiemetics only after symptoms occur

Q354. A patient receiving radiation therapy complains of mouth dryness and altered taste. Which nursing intervention is most effective?
A. Limit fluids before meals
B. Provide salted snacks to increase saliva
C. Offer sugar-free gum and frequent water rinses
D. Encourage mouth rinses with alcohol

Q355. A child receiving chemotherapy develops bruising on arms and legs without trauma. What does this finding indicate?
A. Thrombocytopenia
B. Leukocytosis
C. Hyperbilirubinemia
D. Electrolyte imbalance

Q356. A nurse notes a child receiving doxorubicin has swelling and redness at the IV site. What is the priority nursing action?
A. Stop the infusion and assess for extravasation
B. Apply warm compresses to the site
C. Flush the IV line with saline
D. Reposition the IV catheter

Q357. A patient receiving radiation to the chest area complains of painful swallowing. What nursing recommendation is most appropriate?
A. Restrict oral intake until pain resolves
B. Encourage spicy foods to stimulate appetite
C. Offer citrus juices between meals
D. Provide soft, nonacidic foods and cool liquids

Q358. A child undergoing chemotherapy reports severe mouth pain unrelieved by topical rinses. Which action should the nurse take next?
A. Notify the provider for systemic pain control
B. Encourage carbonated drinks
C. Discontinue oral care temporarily
D. Restrict oral intake to reduce discomfort

Q359. A patient undergoing hematopoietic stem cell transplant develops jaundice and right upper quadrant pain. What should the nurse suspect?
A. Hepatic sinusoidal obstruction syndrome
B. Acute graft-versus-host disease
C. Biliary colic
D. Viral hepatitis

Q360. A nurse is counseling parents of a child receiving chemotherapy about fatigue. Which guidance is most appropriate?
A. Discourage social interactions until therapy completion
B. Avoid all physical activity
C. Increase academic workload to maintain focus
D. Balance activity with rest and encourage short naps

Q361. A child receiving chemotherapy reports severe nausea and vomiting after each treatment. What is the most effective preventive intervention?
A. Administer antiemetics 30 minutes before chemotherapy
B. Offer fluids only after vomiting stops
C. Restrict meals for 12 hours after chemotherapy

D. Encourage the child to eat large meals before therapy

Q362. A child receiving morphine for cancer pain reports itching and mild rash. What is the nurse's best response?

A. Administer prescribed antihistamine and continue monitoring

B. Discontinue morphine immediately

C. Apply ice to the rash area

D. Encourage the child to take a cool shower

Q363. A patient receiving chemotherapy reports painful tingling in the hands and difficulty writing. What should the nurse do first?

A. Apply warm compresses to hands

B. Assess the extent of neuropathy and ensure safety measures

C. Encourage the child to perform fine motor tasks

D. Administer corticosteroids

Q364. A nurse notes a child with a central venous catheter has redness, tenderness, and drainage at the insertion site. What is the priority action?

A. Stop any infusion and obtain a culture of the site

B. Apply heat to the area

C. Continue the infusion and monitor

D. Flush the line with saline

Q365. A child undergoing radiation therapy reports loss of appetite. Which intervention should the nurse nurse recommend?

A. Provide small, nutrient-dense meals and snacks

B. Encourage large meals three times daily

C. Offer strong-flavored foods to stimulate appetite

D. Restrict eating to mealtimes only

Q366. A patient receiving filgrastim (G-CSF) therapy reports bone pain. Which nursing action is most appropriate?

A. Stop the medication immediately

B. Apply heat to affected areas

C. Administer acetaminophen for discomfort

D. Restrict movement of painful areas

Q367. A child on chemotherapy presents with pale skin and tachycardia. What should the nurse suspect?

A. Anemia from bone marrow suppression

B. Hypoglycemia

C. Hypercalcemia

D. Dehydration

Q368. A patient receiving cisplatin reports hearing loss. Which intervention should the nurse anticipate?

A. Schedule audiometric testing and notify the provider

B. Increase IV fluid rate

C. Administer corticosteroids

D. Provide ear drops as ordered

Q369. A child receiving opioids for pain reports constipation despite daily stool softeners. What should the nurse do next?

A. Decrease oral fluid intake

B. Add a stimulant laxative to the regimen

C. Encourage high-protein, low-fiber foods

D. Stop the opioid medication

Q370. A patient with leukemia develops nosebleeds and petechiae. Which safety teaching should the nurse reinforce?

A. Use a soft toothbrush and avoid rough play

B. Engage in normal sports activity

C. Use aspirin for mild headaches

D. Blow the nose forcefully to clear congestion

Q371. A child receiving chemotherapy reports mouth sores and severe pain. What intervention should the nurse initiate first?

A. Assess oral cavity and provide analgesia before meals

B. Encourage citrus fruits for healing

C. Use alcohol-based rinses for cleaning

D. Restrict oral care to once per day

Q372. A patient receiving radiation therapy to the head and neck reports dry mouth and cracked lips. What should the nurse recommend?

A. Eat spicy foods to stimulate saliva

B. Use mouth rinses containing alcohol

C. Restrict fluids between meals

D. Encourage sugar-free gum and frequent water sips

Q373. A child undergoing bone marrow transplant develops diarrhea and abdominal pain. What complication should the nurse suspect?

A. Acute graft-versus-host disease

B. Tumor lysis syndrome
C. Neutropenic enterocolitis
D. Appendicitis

Q374. A nurse notes a child on chemotherapy has an oral temperature of 38.3°C (101°F). What is the immediate action?
A. Notify the provider and initiate blood cultures
B. Administer acetaminophen and reassess
C. Provide cool fluids and rest
D. Recheck temperature in one hour

Q375. A child receiving vincristine therapy reports abdominal pain and lack of bowel movement for five days. What should the nurse suspect?
A. Gastroenteritis
B. Urinary retention
C. Dehydration
D. Paralytic ileus

Q376. A nurse observes that a child undergoing chemotherapy has yellowing of the eyes and skin. What laboratory value should be assessed?
A. Bilirubin level
B. Platelet count
C. Sodium level
D. Blood glucose

Q377. A patient receiving opioids for cancer pain develops respiratory rate of 8/min and pinpoint pupils. What is the priority nursing action?
A. Administer naloxone as prescribed
B. Decrease opioid dose by half
C. Provide oxygen via nasal cannula
D. Encourage deep breathing

Q378. A child receiving chemotherapy develops dry, itchy skin. Which instruction should the nurse provide?
A. Take long baths with bubble soap
B. Apply alcohol-based cleanser daily
C. Use fragrance-free lotion and avoid hot showers
D. Expose skin to sunlight for dryness

Q379. A patient receiving total body irradiation complains of mouth pain, redness, and white patches. What should the nurse suspect?
A. Oral candidiasis
B. Viral stomatitis
C. Gingivitis
D. Chemical burn

Q380. A child undergoing chemotherapy presents with extreme fatigue and irritability. What is the most appropriate nursing intervention?
A. Encourage alternating periods of activity and rest
B. Discourage daytime naps
C. Restrict caloric intake to reduce drowsiness
D. Increase academic workload to maintain focus

Q381. A child receiving doxorubicin develops new-onset shortness of breath and tachycardia. What is the nurse's priority action?
A. Administer diuretics to reduce fluid overload
B. Notify the provider and prepare for cardiac evaluation
C. Reassure the family that fatigue is common
D. Encourage deep breathing exercises

Q382. A child receiving high-dose methotrexate therapy presents with oral ulcers and elevated creatinine. Which intervention should the nurse anticipate?
A. Increased leucovorin rescue and aggressive hydration
B. Administration of corticosteroids
C. Reduction in dietary protein
D. Initiation of diuretics

Q383. A patient receiving vincristine develops foot drop and difficulty walking. What is the appropriate nursing action?
A. Assess gait and provide safety devices for ambulation
B. Increase activity to rebuild muscle strength
C. Apply cold packs to affected muscles
D. Continue therapy without intervention

Q384. A child on a morphine infusion for postoperative pain becomes difficult to arouse and has a respiratory rate of 8/min. What should the nurse do first?
A. Encourage coughing and deep breathing
B. Continue monitoring and reassess in 15 minutes
C. Apply a warm blanket and reduce stimulation
D. Stop the infusion and administer naloxone

Q385. A patient receiving cisplatin reports ringing in the ears and difficulty hearing conversations. What is the most appropriate nursing intervention?

A. Notify the provider and schedule an audiogram
B. Provide ear drops for comfort
C. Reassure the child that symptoms will resolve
D. Increase fluid intake to reduce ototoxicity

Q386. A child receiving radiation to the abdomen reports persistent diarrhea. What is the nurse's best recommendation?
A. Provide a low-residue, lactose-free diet
B. Encourage high-fiber fruits and vegetables
C. Offer spicy foods to stimulate appetite
D. Restrict fluids until stools firm up

Q387. A nurse notes a child with a central venous catheter has redness, tenderness, and purulent drainage at the insertion site. What is the immediate action?
A. Flush the line with saline
B. Apply topical antibiotic ointment
C. Obtain cultures and notify the provider
D. Cover the site with sterile gauze and continue therapy

Q388. A child undergoing chemotherapy reports severe mouth pain and difficulty eating. Which intervention should be prioritized?
A. Administer topical anesthetics before meals
B. Encourage citrus juices for vitamin C
C. Restrict oral intake to reduce pain
D. Offer coarse-textured foods

Q389. A patient undergoing stem cell transplant develops watery diarrhea, rash, and jaundice two weeks after infusion. What complication should the nurse suspect?
A. Acute graft-versus-host disease
B. Sinusoidal obstruction syndrome
C. Neutropenic enterocolitis
D. Viral gastroenteritis

Q390. A nurse caring for a child receiving chemotherapy notices bruising on the arms and legs. What laboratory test is most relevant?
A. Creatinine level
B. White blood cell count
C. Serum calcium
D. Platelet count

Q391. A child with sickle cell disease and leukemia reports chest pain, cough, and fever. What is the nurse's priority action?
A. Administer oxygen and notify the provider immediately
B. Encourage ambulation and deep breathing
C. Provide cough suppressant
D. Apply ice to the chest

Q392. A patient receiving biotherapy develops chills, fever, and rigors during infusion. What is the nurse's first action?
A. Stop the infusion and assess vital signs
B. Administer acetaminophen and continue infusion
C. Slow the infusion rate and reassess
D. Encourage oral hydration

Q393. A nurse observes a patient receiving vincristine has developed a distended abdomen and no bowel movement for several days. Which action should the nurse take?
A. Encourage increased physical activity
B. Administer a strong laxative
C. Report findings as possible paralytic ileus
D. Provide carbonated beverages

Q394. A child on chemotherapy reports fatigue and dizziness. Which laboratory value should be reviewed?
A. Hemoglobin level
B. Serum potassium
C. Blood glucose
D. Sodium level

Q395. A patient receiving corticosteroids for leukemia maintenance reports weight gain and mood swings. What should the nurse include in teaching?
A. Limit salt intake and monitor for behavioral changes
B. Discontinue corticosteroid use immediately
C. Avoid protein in the diet
D. Engage in high-intensity exercise

Q396. A child receiving chemotherapy presents with oral temperature of 38.5°C (101.3°F). What is the immediate nursing action?
A. Recheck temperature in one hour
B. Administer antipyretics immediately
C. Obtain cultures and notify the provider
D. Encourage oral fluids

Q397. A child undergoing radiation therapy develops red, peeling skin in the treatment area. What is the best nursing intervention?
A. Apply gentle, fragrance-free moisturizer
B. Clean the area with alcohol wipes
C. Use adhesive tape for dressings

D. Apply heating pads to relieve discomfort

Q398. A patient receiving chemotherapy complains of persistent headache and visual changes. Which complication should the nurse consider?

A. Increased intracranial pressure from CNS toxicity

B. Hypoglycemia

C. Dehydration

D. Ear infection

Q399. A nurse notices that a child receiving methotrexate has yellow sclera and elevated liver enzymes. What should the nurse anticipate?

A. Increasing the methotrexate dose

B. Holding the medication and notifying the provider

C. Administering leucovorin rescue

D. Providing antiemetics for comfort

Q400. A child with leukemia complains of severe abdominal pain, nausea, and decreased urine output after starting chemotherapy. What complication should the nurse suspect?

A. Tumor lysis syndrome

B. Appendicitis

C. Gastroenteritis

D. Intestinal obstruction

Answer Key and Explanation (301-400)

Q301. Answer: A

Explanation: Chemotherapy can cause dysgeusia, leading to metallic taste and poor appetite. Cold foods and plastic utensils reduce unpleasant flavors by minimizing metal interactions and odor sensitivity. Frequent, small meals support adequate intake.

Subdomain: Nutritional Support – Altered Taste Perception

Q302. Answer: D

Explanation: Agitation or confusion in a patient receiving opioids may signal hypoxia secondary to respiratory depression. Immediate assessment ensures appropriate intervention before administering reversal agents. Prompt oxygen support may stabilize the patient.

Subdomain: Pain Management – Opioid Safety Monitoring

Q303. Answer: A

Explanation: Guided imagery and deep breathing reduce anticipatory anxiety by promoting relaxation and control. These strategies enhance coping and treatment adherence. Emotional support from the healthcare team further reduces distress.

Subdomain: Psychosocial Support – Anxiety Management

Q304. Answer: A

Explanation: Xerostomia from salivary gland damage reduces oral moisture, leading to thick secretions and discomfort. Frequent hydration and sugar-free gum stimulate saliva and maintain mucosal integrity. Alcohol-based rinses worsen dryness.

Subdomain: Oral Symptom Management – Xerostomia

Q305. Answer: B

Explanation: Vincristine causes autonomic neuropathy leading to decreased bowel motility. High-fiber diets and adequate hydration prevent constipation. Regular activity and stool softeners may be used as supportive measures.

Subdomain: Gastrointestinal Symptom Management – Constipation

Q306. Answer: A

Explanation: Thrombocytopenia-related epistaxis requires immediate pressure to control bleeding. Tilting the head forward prevents aspiration of blood. Monitoring for recurrent bleeding and platelet counts guides further management.

Subdomain: Hematologic Supportive Care – Thrombocytopenia

Q307. Answer: A

Explanation: Chemotherapy-induced peripheral neuropathy affects coordination and sensation, increasing fall and injury risk. Safety measures such as nonslip shoes and assistive devices are crucial. Ongoing monitoring ensures timely treatment adjustments.

Subdomain: Neuropathy Management – Safety Precautions

Q308. Answer: D

Explanation: Corticosteroids cause Cushingoid features, increased appetite, and glucose intolerance. Nutritional counseling and regular glucose monitoring help manage side effects. Gradual tapering prevents adrenal insufficiency if discontinuation is required.

Subdomain: Endocrine and Metabolic Symptom Management

Q309. Answer: A

Explanation: Somnolence syndrome is a transient post-radiation effect caused by delayed demyelination. Symptoms include headache, fatigue, and lethargy occurring weeks after therapy. It resolves spontaneously with supportive care.

Subdomain: Neurologic Symptom Management – Radiation Effects

Q310. Answer: A

Explanation: "Chemo brain" or cognitive dysfunction is a common treatment-related effect. Organizational aids, planners, and rest breaks support cognitive functioning. Education and reassurance promote adaptation and reduce frustration.

Subdomain: Cognitive Function Support

Q311. Answer: C

Explanation: Redness and tenderness at a central line site may indicate local or systemic infection. Cultures and prompt antibiotic therapy are necessary to prevent sepsis. Strict

aseptic technique is essential during access and maintenance.
Subdomain: Infection Management – Central Line Care

Q312. Answer: A

Explanation: Vaso-occlusive pain results from ischemia caused by sickled cells. Opioids and heat therapy relieve pain by promoting vasodilation and comfort. Adequate hydration helps reduce sickling episodes.
Subdomain: Pain Management – Hematologic Disorders

Q313. Answer: A

Explanation: Cisplatin can cause ototoxicity due to cochlear hair cell damage, leading to tinnitus and hearing loss. Baseline and serial audiograms help detect toxicity early. Dose adjustments may prevent permanent impairment.
Subdomain: Sensory Symptom Management – Ototoxicity

Q314. Answer: B

Explanation: Graft-versus-host disease occurs when donor T-cells attack host tissues, commonly affecting skin and GI tract. Early detection allows immunosuppressive therapy to limit damage. Ongoing assessment of stool output and rash severity guides treatment.
Subdomain: Immune-Related Symptom Management

Q315. Answer: A

Explanation: Pruritus is a common side effect of opioid therapy caused by histamine release. Antihistamines provide symptom relief without compromising analgesia. Assessment ensures the itching is not due to allergic reaction or infection.
Subdomain: Pain Management – Adverse Effects

Q316. Answer: A

Explanation: Hand-foot syndrome results from capillary damage from certain chemotherapy agents. Avoiding heat, pressure, and friction prevents worsening of symptoms. Emollient creams and protective measures reduce discomfort.
Subdomain: Dermatologic Symptom Management

Q317. Answer: D

Explanation: Pinpoint pupils and respiratory depression indicate opioid toxicity. Immediate administration of naloxone reverses the effects and prevents respiratory arrest. Close monitoring after reversal is necessary due to possible relapse of symptoms.
Subdomain: Pain Management – Opioid Overdose

Q318. Answer: A

Explanation: Consistent bedtime routines support normal circadian rhythm and improve sleep quality. Minimizing screen exposure and caffeine intake further enhances rest. Relaxation strategies also reduce anxiety-related insomnia.
Subdomain: Sleep and Fatigue Management

Q319. Answer: A

Explanation: Radiation-induced esophagitis causes odynophagia, best managed with soft, nonacidic foods and saline rinses. Avoiding irritants prevents worsening of mucosal inflammation. Adequate nutrition and hydration remain priorities.
Subdomain: Gastrointestinal Symptom Management – Esophagitis

Q320. Answer: C

Explanation: Neutropenic patients must avoid raw or unpasteurized foods to minimize infection risk. Cooked and soft foods reduce mucosal irritation while supporting nutrition. Strict food safety education is essential for caregivers.
Subdomain: Infection Prevention – Neutropenic Precautions

Q321. Answer: B

Explanation: Tingling and burning in the extremities indicate peripheral neuropathy, a neurotoxic side effect of agents such as vincristine. Assessing gait and balance ensures safety and prevents injury. Early recognition allows for potential dose adjustments.
Subdomain: Neuropathy Management

Q322. Answer: A

Explanation: Radiation-induced moist desquamation requires nonadherent dressings to protect fragile tissue and prevent infection. Alcohol or heat increases irritation and delays healing. Gentle handling minimizes trauma and promotes comfort.

Subdomain: Dermatologic Symptom Management

Q323. Answer: A

Explanation: Saline rinses soothe mucosal irritation and promote healing in chemotherapy-induced stomatitis. Acidic or peroxide-based products worsen discomfort and delay recovery. Consistent oral care reduces infection risk.

Subdomain: Oral Mucositis Management

Q324. Answer: C

Explanation: Fever in a post-transplant patient may indicate life-threatening infection due to neutropenia. Prompt culture collection and antibiotic initiation are critical. Delay in action increases sepsis risk.

Subdomain: Infection Management – Febrile Neutropenia

Q325. Answer: A

Explanation: Doxorubicin may cause cumulative dose-related cardiomyopathy. Shortness of breath and fatigue are early warning signs of cardiac compromise. Cardiac assessment, including echocardiography, guides management.

Subdomain: Cardiovascular Symptom Management

Q326. Answer: A

Explanation: Small, bland meals minimize gastric irritation and reduce chemotherapy-induced nausea. Maintaining hydration and scheduled antiemetics enhance control of symptoms. Avoiding strong odors further decreases nausea triggers.

Subdomain: Gastrointestinal Symptom Management – Nausea Control

Q327. Answer: D

Explanation: Radiation-induced fatigue is managed through balanced activity and rest schedules. Encouraging energy conservation while maintaining gentle movement prevents deconditioning. Adequate nutrition supports recovery.

Subdomain: Fatigue and Activity Management

Q328. Answer: A

Explanation: Petechiae and bleeding gums suggest thrombocytopenia, a common chemotherapy side effect. Reviewing platelet count determines bleeding risk and transfusion needs. Monitoring oral trauma reduces further complications.

Subdomain: Hematologic Symptom Management

Q329. Answer: A

Explanation: Tinnitus during cisplatin therapy indicates ototoxicity. Reporting promptly and obtaining audiometric assessment allow early dose modification. Preventing permanent hearing loss requires close monitoring.

Subdomain: Sensory Symptom Management – Ototoxicity

Q330. Answer: D

Explanation: Opioid-induced constipation may require a stimulant laxative when stool softeners alone are ineffective. Adequate fluids and activity support bowel motility. Regular assessment ensures effective symptom control.

Subdomain: Gastrointestinal Symptom Management – Constipation

Q331. Answer: A

Explanation: TRALI occurs due to immune-mediated pulmonary capillary leakage following transfusion. Symptoms include dyspnea, hypoxia, and pulmonary infiltrates. Immediate cessation of transfusion and respiratory support are required.

Subdomain: Transfusion Reaction Management

Q332. Answer: A

Explanation: Even mild fever in a neutropenic patient indicates possible sepsis. Immediate cultures and empiric antibiotic therapy reduce mortality risk. Delays can lead to rapid progression of infection.

Subdomain: Infection Management – Neutropenia

Q333. Answer: C

Explanation: Corticosteroids and other agents can cause hyperglycemia, leading to polyuria and polydipsia. Monitoring blood glucose helps detect and manage steroid-induced diabetes early. Dietary and medication adjustments may be required.

Subdomain: Endocrine and Metabolic Management

Q334. Answer: A

Explanation: Cool, soft foods and saline rinses reduce oral discomfort and promote intake in patients with mucositis. Spicy or acidic foods exacerbate pain. Analgesics before meals improve tolerance.

Subdomain: Nutritional Support – Oral Mucositis

Q335. Answer: A

Explanation: Sudden dyspnea during TPN may indicate air embolism from central line disconnection. Stopping infusion and positioning prevent air migration to pulmonary circulation. Emergency oxygen and provider notification follow.

Subdomain: Central Line Complication Management

Q336. Answer: D

Explanation: Neutropenic diets restrict uncooked foods to prevent bacterial exposure. Proper food handling and cooking reduce infection risk. Patients should consume well-cooked meals and bottled fluids.

Subdomain: Infection Prevention – Nutritional Safety

Q337. Answer: A

Explanation: Methotrexate-induced myelosuppression may cause anemia, leading to fatigue. Assessing hemoglobin identifies need for transfusion or supportive care. Balancing rest and mild activity enhances well-being.

Subdomain: Fatigue and Hematologic Support

Q338. Answer: A

Explanation: Peripheral neuropathy impairs fine motor coordination. Adaptive tools and safety strategies prevent injury and promote independence. Reporting progression ensures timely dose evaluation.

Subdomain: Neuropathy Management – Functional Adaptation

Q339. Answer: B

Explanation: Radiation causes temporary alopecia and scalp sensitivity. Gentle cleansing and sun protection maintain comfort and prevent irritation. Emotional reassurance supports body image during regrowth.

Subdomain: Dermatologic and Psychosocial Support

Q340. Answer: A

Explanation: Tumor lysis syndrome results from rapid tumor cell breakdown, leading to uric acid crystallization and renal injury. Monitoring urine output and laboratory values ensures early detection. Aggressive hydration and allopurinol prevent complications.

Subdomain: Metabolic Complication Management

Q341. Answer: A

Explanation: Hematuria and dysuria are signs of hemorrhagic cystitis, a serious toxicity of cyclophosphamide. Prompt reporting, increased hydration, and administration of mesna help protect the bladder. Early intervention prevents long-term complications.

Subdomain: Urologic Symptom Management

Q342. Answer: D

Explanation: Frequent small meals with calorie-dense foods help patients maintain nutrition during therapy-related anorexia. Avoiding food restrictions and optimizing timing of meals enhance intake. Dietitian collaboration ensures balanced nutrition.

Subdomain: Nutritional Support – Anorexia

Q343. Answer: A

Explanation: Thrombocytopenia resulting from bone marrow suppression causes increased bleeding risk, including epistaxis. Reviewing platelet levels determines severity and transfusion needs. Bleeding precautions should be reinforced.

Subdomain: Hematologic Symptom Management

Q344. Answer: A

Explanation: Opioid-induced nausea can be effectively managed with antiemetics and supportive positioning. Routine symptom reassessment ensures proper balance between comfort and side effect control. Adjusting dosage or formulation may be necessary.

Subdomain: Pain Management – Opioid Side Effects

Q345. Answer: C

Explanation: Abdominal radiation can damage intestinal mucosa, causing diarrhea and lactose intolerance. A low-fiber, lactose-free diet reduces bowel stimulation and fluid loss. Gradual reintroduction of foods follows symptom improvement.

Subdomain: Gastrointestinal Symptom Management – Diarrhea

Q346. Answer: A
Explanation: Methotrexate can cause myelosuppression, leading to anemia characterized by low hemoglobin and hematocrit. Fatigue and pallor reflect decreased oxygen delivery. Monitoring counts guides supportive transfusion needs.
Subdomain: Hematologic Supportive Care – Anemia
Q347. Answer: A
Explanation: Oral anesthetics relieve pain and promote nutritional intake in patients with mucositis. Avoiding spicy and alcohol-based products prevents further mucosal injury. Regular mouth care reduces infection risk.
Subdomain: Oral Mucositis Management
Q348. Answer: D
Explanation: High-dose cytarabine can cause cerebellar toxicity manifesting as confusion, slurred speech, and ataxia. Immediate cessation of chemotherapy prevents permanent damage. Neurologic assessments are critical during therapy.
Subdomain: Neurologic Symptom Management
Q349. Answer: A
Explanation: Infusion reactions are common during biotherapy due to cytokine release. Stopping the infusion and assessing the patient's stability prevent progression to anaphylaxis. Subsequent management may include antipyretics or corticosteroids.
Subdomain: Biotherapy – Infusion Reaction Management
Q350. Answer: A
Explanation: Vincristine causes autonomic neuropathy leading to decreased bowel motility. A combination of stool softeners and mild stimulants promotes regular elimination. Hydration and diet modifications further prevent recurrence.
Subdomain: Gastrointestinal Symptom Management – Constipation
Q351. Answer: B
Explanation: Acute chest syndrome results from sickled cells obstructing pulmonary vessels, leading to inflammation and hypoxia. Immediate evaluation, oxygen, and antibiotics are needed. It is a life-threatening complication requiring rapid intervention.
Subdomain: Pulmonary Symptom Management
Q352. Answer: A
Explanation: Filgrastim stimulates bone marrow activity, commonly causing bone pain. Acetaminophen relieves discomfort without interfering with the drug's action. Persistent pain may warrant dose evaluation.
Subdomain: Supportive Care – Growth Factor Therapy
Q353. Answer: A
Explanation: Preemptive antiemetic therapy blocks neurotransmitter activation before chemotherapy, preventing anticipatory nausea. Combining behavioral and pharmacologic interventions maximizes control. Consistency improves treatment tolerance.
Subdomain: Nausea and Vomiting – Preventive Care
Q354. Answer: C
Explanation: Xerostomia from radiation therapy requires hydration and saliva stimulation through sugar-free gum or rinses. Avoiding irritants maintains comfort and oral health. Good oral hygiene reduces secondary infections.
Subdomain: Oral Symptom Management – Xerostomia
Q355. Answer: A
Explanation: Spontaneous bruising signals low platelet count due to chemotherapy-induced myelosuppression. Monitoring laboratory values and bleeding signs guides care. Precautionary measures reduce injury risk.
Subdomain: Hematologic Supportive Care
Q356. Answer: A
Explanation: Doxorubicin is a vesicant, and extravasation can cause severe tissue necrosis. Stopping the infusion immediately limits exposure. Cold compresses and antidote administration may be required.
Subdomain: Chemotherapy Administration – Extravasation Management
Q357. Answer: D
Explanation: Esophagitis from chest radiation benefits from soft, nonacidic foods and cool fluids. This approach reduces irritation and

maintains caloric intake. Analgesics may be prescribed for additional comfort.
Subdomain: Gastrointestinal Symptom Management – Esophagitis

Q358. Answer: A

Explanation: Severe mucositis pain may require systemic analgesics for adequate relief. Effective pain control promotes nutritional intake and healing. Ongoing oral hygiene remains critical to prevent infection.
Subdomain: Pain and Oral Care Management

Q359. Answer: A

Explanation: Sinusoidal obstruction syndrome results from hepatic venule injury after high-dose chemotherapy or radiation. It presents with jaundice, weight gain, and hepatomegaly. Early recognition allows prompt supportive management.
Subdomain: Hepatic Symptom Management

Q360. Answer: D

Explanation: Chemotherapy-related fatigue improves with balanced activity and rest. Encouraging mild physical activity and structured rest promotes energy conservation. Psychosocial engagement supports overall well-being.
Subdomain: Fatigue and Coping Support

Q361. Answer: A

Explanation: Administering antiemetics before chemotherapy prevents activation of nausea pathways and enhances comfort. Early prophylaxis reduces both acute and anticipatory symptoms. Combining medication with relaxation techniques maximizes relief.
Subdomain: Gastrointestinal Symptom Management – Nausea and Vomiting

Q362. Answer: A

Explanation: Mild pruritus is a common morphine side effect due to histamine release. Antihistamines relieve itching without reducing analgesic efficacy. Close monitoring ensures the reaction is not progressing to hypersensitivity.
Subdomain: Pain Management – Opioid Side Effects

Q363. Answer: B

Explanation: Neuropathy affects coordination and safety; assessing functional status allows appropriate precautions and early reporting. Dose adjustment may prevent worsening of symptoms. Occupational therapy can support adaptation.
Subdomain: Neuropathy Management – Safety and Assessment

Q364. Answer: A

Explanation: Redness and drainage at a central line site indicate possible infection. Stopping infusion and obtaining cultures ensures early identification of pathogens. Prompt antibiotics prevent systemic sepsis.
Subdomain: Infection Management – Central Line Care

Q365. Answer: A

Explanation: Radiation-related anorexia is best managed with small, frequent meals rich in protein and calories. Gentle encouragement and appealing food presentation improve intake. Nutritional counseling supports growth and recovery.
Subdomain: Nutritional Support – Appetite Management

Q366. Answer: C

Explanation: Filgrastim stimulates bone marrow, often causing bone pain due to increased marrow activity. Acetaminophen effectively manages symptoms without interfering with therapy. Monitoring pain trends ensures tolerability.
Subdomain: Supportive Care – Growth Factor Therapy

Q367. Answer: A

Explanation: Pallor and tachycardia are signs of anemia due to chemotherapy-induced marrow suppression. Low red blood cell count decreases oxygen delivery to tissues. Blood transfusion or erythropoietin therapy may be indicated.
Subdomain: Hematologic Supportive Care – Anemia

Q368. Answer: A

Explanation: Ototoxicity is a known cisplatin side effect that can cause permanent hearing damage. Audiometry confirms severity, guiding dose adjustment or discontinuation. Early monitoring prevents irreversible loss.
Subdomain: Sensory Symptom Management – Ototoxicity

Q369. Answer: B

Explanation: Opioid-induced constipation may require both stool softeners and stimulant laxatives to promote bowel movement. Hydration and physical activity enhance effectiveness. Continued monitoring prevents discomfort and impaction.
Subdomain: Gastrointestinal Symptom Management – Constipation

Q370. Answer: A

Explanation: Thrombocytopenia increases bleeding risk; using soft oral care tools and limiting injury-prone activities prevent hemorrhage. Aspirin and other anticoagulants must be avoided. Education ensures consistent safety practices.
Subdomain: Hematologic Symptom Management – Bleeding Precautions

Q371. Answer: A

Explanation: Painful mucositis requires timely pain control and gentle assessment to maintain nutrition and hydration. Citrus and alcohol irritants exacerbate injury. Regular saline rinses support healing.
Subdomain: Oral Mucositis and Pain Management

Q372. Answer: D

Explanation: Xerostomia from radiation reduces salivary flow, leading to dryness and discomfort. Sugar-free gum stimulates saliva production, while hydration maintains mucosal moisture. Alcohol-based products worsen dryness and should be avoided.
Subdomain: Oral Symptom Management – Xerostomia

Q373. Answer: A

Explanation: Acute graft-versus-host disease often manifests with diarrhea, rash, and liver dysfunction after transplant. Early immunosuppressive therapy prevents severe systemic involvement. Continuous monitoring for dehydration is essential.
Subdomain: Immune-Related Symptom Management

Q374. Answer: A

Explanation: Any fever in an immunocompromised child indicates possible neutropenic infection. Rapid culture collection and antibiotic administration are life-saving measures. Delays can lead to septic shock.
Subdomain: Infection Management – Febrile Neutropenia

Q375. Answer: D

Explanation: Vincristine causes autonomic neuropathy that may lead to paralytic ileus, presenting with abdominal distension and constipation. Immediate reporting allows dose adjustment and bowel rest. Monitoring bowel sounds ensures safety.
Subdomain: Gastrointestinal Symptom Management – Neurotoxicity

Q376. Answer: A

Explanation: Elevated bilirubin indicates hepatotoxicity, a potential side effect of many chemotherapeutic agents. Monitoring liver function ensures early detection and dose modification. Supportive care prevents progression to hepatic failure.
Subdomain: Hepatic Symptom Management

Q377. Answer: A

Explanation: Respiratory depression with miosis signals opioid overdose. Immediate administration of naloxone reverses effects and prevents respiratory arrest. Continuous monitoring ensures stabilization.
Subdomain: Pain Management – Opioid Toxicity

Q378. Answer: C

Explanation: Chemotherapy can cause xerosis and pruritus; gentle skin care with fragrance-free moisturizers helps maintain barrier function. Avoiding hot water prevents further dryness. Consistent hydration supports skin health.
Subdomain: Integumentary Symptom Management

Q379. Answer: A

Explanation: Immunosuppression from radiation predisposes patients to fungal infections such as oral candidiasis. Symptoms include erythema and white plaques on mucosa. Antifungal agents and good oral hygiene are essential.
Subdomain: Infection Management – Oral Fungal Infections

Q380. Answer: A

Explanation: Fatigue is common during chemotherapy and improves with structured rest balanced by light activity. Maintaining routines helps prevent deconditioning and supports emotional stability. Family education ensures consistency at home.

Subdomain: Fatigue and Coping Support

Q381. Answer: B

Explanation: Doxorubicin can cause dose-dependent cardiotoxicity due to myocardial cell injury. Early symptoms include dyspnea, fatigue, and tachycardia. Prompt evaluation with echocardiography ensures early intervention and prevents cardiac failure.

Subdomain: Cardiovascular Symptom Management – Anthracycline Toxicity

Q382. Answer: A

Explanation: Elevated creatinine indicates delayed methotrexate clearance, increasing mucosal and renal toxicity risk. Intensified leucovorin rescue and hydration promote drug elimination. Monitoring urine pH ensures alkalinization for renal protection.

Subdomain: Renal and Mucosal Symptom Management

Q383. Answer: A

Explanation: Vincristine-induced peripheral neuropathy may manifest as foot drop and motor weakness. Safety assessment and use of supportive devices prevent injury. Reporting symptoms early helps guide dose modification.

Subdomain: Neuromuscular Symptom Management – Chemotherapy-Induced Neuropathy

Q384. Answer: D

Explanation: Sedation and respiratory depression are signs of opioid overdose. Immediate discontinuation and naloxone administration reverse respiratory compromise. Continuous monitoring ensures patient safety after reversal.

Subdomain: Pain Management – Opioid Toxicity Response

Q385. Answer: A

Explanation: Cisplatin causes cochlear hair cell damage leading to irreversible hearing loss if unaddressed. Early audiologic testing identifies threshold changes for treatment modification. Baseline and serial assessments are standard practice.

Subdomain: Sensory Symptom Management – Ototoxicity

Q386. Answer: A

Explanation: Radiation damages intestinal mucosa, causing malabsorption and lactose intolerance. A low-residue, lactose-free diet reduces irritation and stool frequency. Adequate hydration prevents dehydration.

Subdomain: Gastrointestinal Symptom Management – Radiation Enteritis

Q387. Answer: C

Explanation: Redness and drainage indicate a possible line infection, which can rapidly progress to sepsis in immunocompromised patients. Cultures guide targeted antibiotic therapy. Early intervention reduces systemic risk.

Subdomain: Infection Management – Central Line Care

Q388. Answer: A

Explanation: Oral mucositis requires adequate pain management to maintain nutrition and comfort. Topical anesthetics or systemic analgesics relieve discomfort before meals. Gentle oral hygiene reduces infection risk.

Subdomain: Oral Mucositis and Pain Control

Q389. Answer: A

Explanation: Acute GVHD occurs when donor lymphocytes attack host tissues, primarily the skin, liver, and gastrointestinal tract. Early recognition allows initiation of immunosuppressive therapy to limit progression.

Subdomain: Immune-Related Complications

Q390. Answer: D

Explanation: Bruising without trauma suggests thrombocytopenia due to bone marrow suppression. Monitoring platelet count determines bleeding risk and transfusion needs. Preventive teaching focuses on minimizing injury.

Subdomain: Hematologic Symptom Management – Thrombocytopenia

Q391. Answer: A

Explanation: These symptoms suggest acute chest syndrome, a life-threatening vaso-occlusive complication. Prompt oxygen administration, hydration, and antibiotics are

required. Rapid response prevents respiratory failure.
Subdomain: Pulmonary Symptom Management – Sickle Cell Crisis

Q392. Answer: A
Explanation: Infusion reactions during biotherapy can escalate quickly to severe cytokine release or anaphylaxis. Stopping the infusion and assessing stability ensures safety. Supportive medications and slower rates may be used later.
Subdomain: Biotherapy Symptom Management – Infusion Reactions

Q393. Answer: C
Explanation: Vincristine can cause autonomic neuropathy leading to paralytic ileus. Reporting promptly allows provider evaluation and cessation of therapy if needed. Supportive management prevents bowel perforation.
Subdomain: Gastrointestinal Symptom Management – Neurotoxicity

Q394. Answer: A
Explanation: Fatigue and dizziness indicate anemia secondary to bone marrow suppression. Reviewing hemoglobin confirms need for transfusion or further evaluation. Supportive rest and nutrition help manage symptoms.
Subdomain: Fatigue and Hematologic Support

Q395. Answer: A
Explanation: Corticosteroids cause sodium retention and emotional lability. Education on sodium reduction, glucose monitoring, and gradual tapering supports long-term safety. Family awareness helps identify early behavioral effects.
Subdomain: Endocrine and Metabolic Symptom Management

Q396. Answer: C
Explanation: Fever in a neutropenic patient requires immediate evaluation for infection. Blood cultures and broad-spectrum antibiotics are initiated rapidly. Early action prevents septic progression.
Subdomain: Infection Management – Neutropenic Fever

Q397. Answer: A
Explanation: Radiation dermatitis requires gentle care with mild, fragrance-free moisturizers. Avoiding irritants like alcohol or adhesives prevents further damage. Skin protection education promotes healing.
Subdomain: Integumentary Symptom Management – Radiation Dermatitis

Q398. Answer: A
Explanation: Some chemotherapeutic agents can cross the blood-brain barrier, causing CNS toxicity. Headache and vision changes suggest increased intracranial pressure. Immediate evaluation prevents neurologic deterioration.
Subdomain: Neurologic Symptom Management – CNS Toxicity

Q399. Answer: B
Explanation: Hepatotoxicity is a known side effect of methotrexate, evidenced by jaundice and increased transaminases. Withholding the drug and notifying the provider prevent further liver damage. Ongoing monitoring ensures recovery.
Subdomain: Hepatic Symptom Management – Chemotherapy Toxicity

Q400. Answer: A
Explanation: Tumor lysis syndrome results from rapid tumor breakdown, leading to elevated uric acid, potassium, and phosphate levels. Symptoms include flank pain and oliguria. Immediate hydration and allopurinol prevent renal failure.
Subdomain: Metabolic Emergency Management – Tumor Lysis Syndrome

Question (401-500)

Q401. A child receiving ifosfamide develops confusion and hallucinations during treatment. What is the nurse's priority action?

A. Stop the infusion and notify the provider immediately

B. Administer antiemetics and continue therapy

C. Encourage oral fluids to promote excretion

D. Provide reassurance to the family

Q402. A patient undergoing radiation therapy to the abdomen reports nausea before each session. Which nursing strategy best prevents anticipatory nausea?

A. Offer spicy foods to distract from nausea

B. Combine antiemetics with relaxation techniques before treatment

C. Increase fiber intake before each session

D. Avoid all oral intake for 12 hours before therapy

Q403. A nurse observes a child with mucositis has thick secretions and foul breath. What is the best nursing intervention?

A. Encourage frequent saline rinses and soft toothbrush use

B. Provide alcohol-based mouthwash twice daily

C. Restrict oral intake until symptoms improve

D. Offer citrus juices for vitamin C

Q404. A child receiving corticosteroid therapy for leukemia maintenance has facial rounding and mood swings. What should the nurse teach the family?

A. These effects are temporary and reversible after tapering

B. Stop the medication if mood changes worsen

C. Double the dose on alternate days

D. Restrict protein in the diet

Q405. A patient receiving chemotherapy develops tingling in the fingers and toes. What is the priority nursing assessment?

A. Check for dehydration

B. Encourage hand exercises to promote circulation

C. Apply warm compresses to extremities

D. Evaluate motor strength and ability to perform fine tasks

Q406. A child receiving total parenteral nutrition (TPN) suddenly develops shortness of breath and chest pain. What should the nurse suspect?

A. Air embolism

B. Anxiety

C. Fluid overload

D. Pulmonary infection

Q407. A patient receiving methotrexate complains of extreme fatigue and pallor. Which laboratory value is most relevant to review?

A. Hemoglobin level

B. Serum calcium

C. White blood cell count

D. Potassium level

Q408. A child receiving radiation to the head and neck develops painful swallowing and oral ulcers. Which nursing intervention is appropriate?

A. Apply topical anesthetic only after meals

B. Offer acidic fruit juices for hydration

C. Provide soft, bland foods and saline mouth rinses

D. Encourage dry, crunchy foods for texture

Q409. A child receiving high-dose cytarabine develops confusion and ataxia. What should the nurse do first?

A. Stop the infusion and notify the provider

B. Encourage oral hydration

C. Document findings and continue therapy

D. Administer antiemetics

Q410. A patient undergoing chemotherapy develops jaundice and elevated liver enzymes. What is the nurse's best action?

A. Hold the next chemotherapy dose and notify the provider

B. Encourage high-protein meals

C. Administer corticosteroids

D. Continue treatment with increased hydration

Q411. A child receiving biotherapy develops chills and fever shortly after infusion begins. What should the nurse do first?

A. Continue infusion at a slower rate.

B. Administer antihistamines immediately

C. Reassure the child that chills are expected

D. Stop the infusion and assess vital signs

Q412. A patient receiving cyclophosphamide reports pain on urination. What nursing intervention is essential?

A. Increase hydration and encourage frequent voiding
B. Apply cold compresses to the abdomen
C. Restrict fluids to minimize bladder irritation
D. Delay urination to reduce urgency

Q413. A child receiving radiation therapy develops dry, peeling skin at the treatment site. What should the nurse recommend?

A. Apply nonirritating, fragrance-free moisturizer
B. Wash the area with alcohol wipes
C. Use tight clothing over the area
D. Apply adhesive dressings

Q414. A nurse observes that a child undergoing chemotherapy is withdrawn and avoids social interactions. What is the best intervention?

A. Provide additional sedation for rest
B. Limit visitors to reduce overstimulation
C. Encourage participation in age-appropriate activities
D. Focus on physical symptoms only

Q415. A child undergoing bone marrow transplant develops jaundice, weight gain, and right upper quadrant pain. What complication should the nurse suspect?

A. Hepatic sinusoidal obstruction syndrome
B. Acute graft-versus-host disease
C. Viral hepatitis
D. Pancreatitis

Q416. A patient receiving chemotherapy reports nosebleeds and petechiae. What education should the nurse provide?

A. Avoid rough play and use soft toothbrushes
B. Perform vigorous oral care daily
C. Increase iron-rich foods
D. Take aspirin for mild headaches

Q417. A child receiving methotrexate complains of severe mouth sores and bleeding gums. Which nursing intervention is most appropriate?

A. Offer acidic beverages to cleanse the mouth
B. Provide saline mouth rinses and topical anesthetics
C. Brush with a firm toothbrush twice daily
D. Apply peroxide rinse after each meal

Q418. A child receiving vincristine therapy reports inability to lift the foot when walking. What should the nurse do first?

A. Notify the provider and assess for neuropathy progression
B. Encourage ambulation for muscle strengthening
C. Apply warm compresses to the calf
D. Continue chemotherapy as scheduled

Q419. A patient receiving morphine for cancer pain develops shallow breathing and oxygen saturation of 88%. What is the nurse's priority action?

A. Administer naloxone per protocol
B. Encourage deep breathing
C. Decrease morphine dose by half
D. Provide oxygen and continue monitoring

Q420. A child receiving chemotherapy develops muscle cramps, confusion, and cardiac arrhythmia. What complication should the nurse suspect?

A. Septic shock
B. Dehydration
C. Tumor lysis syndrome
D. Hypoglycemia

Q421. A child receiving high-dose methotrexate develops decreased urine output and flank pain. What should the nurse suspect?

A. Methotrexate-induced nephrotoxicity
B. Tumor lysis syndrome
C. Hypovolemic shock
D. Urinary tract infection

Q422. A child on chemotherapy presents with persistent cough, fever, and dyspnea. What complication should the nurse suspect?

A. Pneumocystis jirovecii pneumonia
B. Upper respiratory infection
C. Bronchitis
D. Pleural effusion

Q423. A patient receiving biotherapy develops severe hypotension, tachycardia, and high fever. What should the nurse do first?

A. Slow the infusion rate and monitor
B. Stop the infusion and initiate emergency management
C. Administer acetaminophen and reassess
D. Apply cool compresses to the forehead

Q424. A child undergoing radiation therapy develops thick saliva and difficulty swallowing. What is the most appropriate nursing recommendation?

A. Encourage frequent sips of water and oral rinses
B. Offer acidic beverages to thin secretions
C. Limit oral fluids between meals
D. Provide dry snacks for texture

Q425. A patient receiving vincristine reports constipation and abdominal distension. Which nursing action is most appropriate?
A. Initiate bowel regimen with stool softener and mild stimulant
B. Restrict oral fluids to prevent bloating
C. Encourage high-protein, low-fiber diet
D. Delay bowel care until chemotherapy completion

Q426. A child receiving morphine for postoperative pain develops nausea and vomiting. What nursing intervention is most effective?
A. Restrict all oral intake
B. Discontinue morphine immediately
C. Offer carbonated beverages
D. Administer prescribed antiemetic and reassess response

Q427. A nurse is caring for a child receiving anthracycline therapy who reports shortness of breath during mild activity. What should the nurse anticipate?
A. Evaluation for possible cardiomyopathy
B. Administration of fluids for dehydration
C. Increase in antiemetic therapy
D. Initiation of antibiotics

Q428. A child undergoing hematopoietic stem cell transplant develops a diffuse rash, diarrhea, and elevated bilirubin. What is the likely cause?
A. Acute graft-versus-host disease
B. Viral gastroenteritis
C. Sinusoidal obstruction syndrome
D. Allergic drug reaction

Q429. A patient receiving chemotherapy reports tingling in the hands and difficulty buttoning clothes. Which intervention should the nurse prioritize?
A. Encourage increased exercise to restore function
B. Assess for neuropathy and ensure safety with ADLs
C. Provide heat therapy for comfort
D. Continue therapy without modification

Q430. A nurse observes petechiae and minor nosebleeds in a child undergoing chemotherapy. What should be included in the care plan?
A. Avoid rectal temperatures and invasive procedures
B. Encourage active play for circulation
C. Use hard toothbrushes for oral hygiene
D. Administer aspirin for pain relief

Q431. A child receiving chemotherapy presents with fever, tachycardia, and hypotension. Blood cultures are drawn and broad-spectrum antibiotics are initiated. What is the nurse's highest priority intervention?
A. Begin intravenous fluid resuscitation
B. Obtain urine for culture and sensitivity
C. Administer colony-stimulating factors
D. Apply warm blankets for comfort

Q432. A neutropenic child develops abdominal pain, fever, and right lower quadrant tenderness. What nursing action is most appropriate?
A. Administer stool softeners as prescribed
B. Encourage ambulation and oral fluids
C. Notify the provider immediately and withhold oral intake
D. Apply warm compresses to the abdomen

Q433. A child receiving induction chemotherapy for leukemia develops hyperuricemia, hyperkalemia, and hypocalcemia. Which intervention should the nurse anticipate?
A. Aggressive IV hydration and administration of allopurinol
B. Fluid restriction and administration of calcium supplements
C. IV potassium chloride replacement
D. Administration of packed red blood cells

Q434. A patient with acute promyelocytic leukemia develops bleeding from venipuncture sites and decreasing fibrinogen levels. What should the nurse prepare to administer?
A. Fresh frozen plasma and cryoprecipitate
B. Heparin infusion
C. Desmopressin nasal spray
D. Platelet inhibitors

Q435. An adolescent with a mediastinal mass reports shortness of breath when lying flat. What should the nurse do first?
A. Place the patient supine for comfort
B. Sit the patient upright to ease breathing
C. Administer bronchodilator therapy
D. Encourage deep breathing and coughing

Q436. A child with a brain tumor has headache, vomiting without nausea, and irritability. What should the nurse do?
A. Elevate the head of bed to 30 degrees
B. Place the child in Trendelenburg position
C. Encourage oral fluids
D. Encourage coughing exercises

Q437. A child on vincristine therapy presents with hyponatremia, weight gain, and low urine output. Which intervention should the nurse anticipate?
A. Fluid restriction and close monitoring of electrolytes
B. Increase IV fluids to maintain urine output
C. Administer oral sodium supplements freely
D. Restrict dietary sodium intake

Q438. A child with sickle cell disease presents with respiratory distress, fever, and chest pain. What complication does the nurse suspect?
A. Pneumothorax
B. Pulmonary embolism
C. Pleural effusion
D. Acute chest syndrome

Q439. A child undergoing treatment for leukemia experiences seizures and blurred vision. Blood pressure is elevated, and MRI shows white matter changes. What condition is likely?
A. Posterior reversible encephalopathy syndrome
B. Intracranial hemorrhage
C. Spinal cord compression
D. Brain metastasis

Q440. A child with sickle cell anemia presents with rapidly enlarging spleen and falling hematocrit. What is the immediate nursing priority?
A. Prepare for emergent transfusion
B. Apply warm compresses to abdomen
C. Encourage oral hydration
D. Position child flat for comfort

Q441. A child with leukemia develops severe left upper quadrant pain, jaundice, and ascites after stem cell transplant. The nurse suspects which complication?
A. Nephrotic syndrome
B. Acute pancreatitis
C. Sinusoidal obstructive syndrome
D. Cholecystitis

Q442. A child with hemophilia reports sudden joint pain and swelling after minor trauma. What nursing action is indicated?
A. Immobilize the joint and apply ice
B. Encourage ambulation
C. Perform range-of-motion exercises
D. Apply warm compresses immediately

Q443. A child with neuroblastoma has severe hypertension and tachycardia during tumor manipulation. The nurse recognizes this as likely caused by:
A. Catecholamine release
B. Hypovolemia
C. Allergic reaction
D. Anesthetic overdose

Q444. A patient receiving asparaginase develops sudden wheezing, hypotension, and hives. What is the nurse's immediate action?
A. Slow the infusion rate
B. Stop the infusion and maintain airway
C. Flush the line and observe for changes
D. Document findings and continue therapy

Q445. During chemotherapy administration, a nurse notes pain and swelling at the IV site with erythema extending along the vein. What is the initial action?
A. Stop the infusion immediately
B. Apply warm compresses and continue therapy
C. Inject saline to dilute the medication
D. Elevate the limb and continue observation

Q446. A patient undergoing high-dose methotrexate therapy presents with confusion and oliguria. What is the nurse's first priority?
A. Assess urine pH and continue leucovorin rescue
B. Administer diuretics to increase urine output
C. Encourage oral hydration
D. Delay next methotrexate dose only

Q447. A child with sickle cell disease presents with severe limb pain unrelieved by standard analgesics. What should the nurse assess next?
A. Blood glucose levels
B. Capillary refill only
C. Hydration status and oxygen saturation
D. Heart rhythm
Q448. After hematopoietic stem cell transplant, a child develops fever, rash, and diarrhea. What complication should the nurse suspect?
A. Graft-versus-host disease
B. Cytokine release syndrome
C. Tumor lysis syndrome
D. Allergic reaction
Q449. A child receiving CAR-T cell therapy develops fever, hypotension, and hypoxia within 48 hours. What is the priority nursing action?
A. Notify provider and initiate cytokine release management protocol
B. Start broad-spectrum antibiotics immediately
C. Administer antihistamines for allergic reaction
D. Encourage oral fluids
Q450. A patient on total parenteral nutrition after abdominal surgery for tumor removal suddenly presents with abdominal distension and vomiting. What is the nurse's initial concern?
A. Peritonitis
B. Bowel obstruction
C. Pancreatitis
D. Gastritis
Q451. A child with acute lymphoblastic leukemia develops fever, hypotension, and delayed capillary refill. The nurse initiates antibiotics. What additional action should occur immediately?
A. Begin oxygen therapy
B. Obtain chest radiograph
C. Administer IV fluid bolus
D. Assess for pain
Q452. A neutropenic child receiving chemotherapy reports severe abdominal cramping and diarrhea. What is the nurse's priority action?
A. Administer stool softeners
B. Obtain stool cultures
C. Notify provider and stop oral intake
D. Encourage clear fluids
Q453. A child with leukemia develops shortness of breath and cough. Chest X-ray reveals pulmonary infiltrates. Which finding requires the nurse's most urgent response?
A. Mild crackles on auscultation
B. Oxygen saturation of 84%
C. White blood cell count of 5,000/mm^3
D. Dry cough with low-grade fever
Q454. During platelet transfusion, a child develops chills, fever, and urticaria. What is the nurse's first action?
A. Slow the transfusion rate
B. Administer acetaminophen
C. Stop the transfusion immediately
D. Obtain a urine specimen
Q455. A child with acute myeloid leukemia is receiving cytarabine and develops hyperglycemia, confusion, and tachypnea. Which laboratory value supports the suspected diagnosis of metabolic acidosis?
A. pH 7.25
B. pH 7.45
C. HCO_3^- 26 mEq/L
D. $PaCO_2$ 45 mm Hg
Q456. After hematopoietic stem cell transplant, a child presents with fever, hypotension, and hypoxia. The nurse suspects cytokine release syndrome. Which medication should be anticipated?
A. Tocilizumab
B. Epinephrine
C. Allopurinol
D. Vancomycin
Q457. A child receiving chemotherapy has blood pressure 80/40 mmHg, heart rate 150, and poor perfusion. Despite two fluid boluses, perfusion remains poor. What is the next intervention?
A. Administer dopamine infusion
B. Begin diuretic therapy
C. Give antihypertensive medication
D. Increase fluid rate further
Q458. A child with sickle cell disease complains of abdominal pain, pallor, and an enlarged spleen. Which intervention takes priority?
A. Administer opioid for pain
B. Prepare for immediate transfusion

C. Encourage oral hydration
D. Apply warm compress to abdomen

Q459. A child receiving vincristine reports muscle weakness and difficulty walking. What should the nurse do next?
A. Notify provider of possible neurotoxicity
B. Encourage ambulation for strength
C. Administer diuretics to reduce swelling
D. Provide electrolyte replacement

Q460. A child with sickle cell disease develops sudden chest pain, dyspnea, and fever. Chest X-ray reveals new infiltrates. Which treatment should the nurse anticipate first?
A. Oxygen therapy and antibiotics
B. Corticosteroids and hydration
C. Analgesics and antihistamines
D. Bronchodilator therapy only

Q461. After CAR-T cell infusion, a child exhibits confusion and seizures. The nurse suspects neurotoxicity. What is the first nursing action?
A. Notify school nurse of event.
B. Administer antihypertensive medication
C. Start IV dextrose
D. Ensure airway and safety measures

Q462. A child receiving chemotherapy suddenly complains of flank pain and hematuria. Which condition should the nurse suspect?
A. Hemorrhagic cystitis
B. Pyelonephritis
C. Nephrotic syndrome
D. Ureteral obstruction

Q463. A patient with leukemia presents with confusion and headache. Labs show WBC count >200,000/mm^3. What should the nurse anticipate?
A. Initiation of leukapheresis
B. Administration of platelet transfusion
C. Increase in corticosteroid dose
D. Start of radiation therapy

Q464. A patient with sickle cell disease reports severe pain in joints and chest. Which nursing intervention best supports physiologic recovery?
A. Apply cold packs to painful areas
B. Restrict fluids to prevent overload
C. Administer IV fluids and oxygen
D. Encourage rest without hydration

Q465. After hematopoietic stem cell transplant, a patient develops jaundice, painful hepatomegaly, and ascites. Which condition does the nurse suspect?
A. Sinusoidal obstructive syndrome
B. Tumor lysis syndrome
C. Graft rejection
D. Sepsis

Q466. A child with leukemia develops severe headache and double vision. Which finding requires urgent action?
A. Papilledema
B. Slight dizziness
C. Decreased appetite
D. Nasal congestion

Q467. A patient undergoing chemotherapy develops confusion and tetany. Labs show calcium 6.2 mg/dL, phosphorus 8.5 mg/dL. What is the likely cause?
A. Diabetes insipidus
B. Tumor lysis syndrome
C. SIADH
D. Hepatic failure

Q468. A child with leukemia on high-dose steroids presents with severe abdominal pain and elevated amylase. What condition should the nurse suspect?
A. Pancreatitis
B. Bowel obstruction
C. Appendicitis
D. Typhlitis

Q469. A child receiving chemotherapy suddenly becomes unresponsive. Pulse and respirations are absent. What is the nurse's immediate action?
A. Initiate cardiopulmonary resuscitation
B. Administer oxygen via nasal cannula
C. Notify family immediately
D. Start IV fluids

Q470. A child receiving ifosfamide develops confusion and seizures. The nurse recognizes this as a manifestation of:
A. Tumor lysis syndrome
B. Brain metastasis
C. Drug-induced encephalopathy
D. SIADH

Q471. A child undergoing induction chemotherapy for leukemia develops oliguria

and hyperkalemia. What is the nurse's immediate priority?
A. Begin potassium replacement therapy
B. Notify the provider and prepare for dialysis
C. Encourage oral fluid intake
D. Restrict IV fluids

Q472. A patient with sickle cell disease reports acute chest pain, cough, and low oxygen saturation. What is the initial nursing intervention?
A. Start oxygen and notify the provider
B. Administer antihistamines
C. Position the patient supine
D. Encourage ambulation to expand lungs

Q473. A child receiving cyclophosphamide reports dysuria and hematuria. What nursing action is indicated?
A. Encourage fluid restriction
B. Discontinue hydration and give antiemetics
C. Continue IV hydration and notify the provider
D. Apply heat packs for comfort

Q474. A patient post–stem cell transplant develops jaundice, hepatomegaly, and rapid weight gain. Which intervention should the nurse anticipate?
A. Administering defibrotide
B. Increasing fluid intake
C. Restricting protein
D. Providing corticosteroids

Q475. During chemotherapy infusion, a child suddenly experiences facial flushing, dyspnea, and hypotension. What is the nurse's first action?
A. Record vital signs and continue slowly
B. Administer corticosteroids
C. Notify provider after completing infusion
D. Stop the infusion and assess airway

Q476. A child with sickle cell anemia presents with severe pallor, fatigue, and an enlarged spleen. Laboratory results show decreased hemoglobin and hematocrit. What is the appropriate nursing action?
A. Prepare for emergent red blood cell transfusion
B. Encourage ambulation to reduce splenic congestion
C. Administer diuretics
D. Begin corticosteroid therapy

Q477. A child receiving high-dose cytarabine develops sudden confusion and ataxia. What is the nurse's best response?
A. Notify the provider and hold the medication
B. Continue therapy with close observation
C. Encourage ambulation for balance
D. Administer antihistamines for side effects

Q478. A child with acute myeloid leukemia reports sudden shortness of breath and decreased breath sounds on one side after central line placement. What is the nurse's immediate action?
A. Apply warm compress to insertion site
B. Reposition the child for comfort
C. Administer diuretics
D. Notify the provider and prepare for chest decompression

Q479. A child with leukemia has a fever and WBC count of 200,000/mm^3. The nurse recognizes the risk for which complication?
A. Stroke
B. Thrombocytopenia
C. Neutropenia
D. Hyponatremia

Q480. A child with sickle cell disease presents with persistent priapism lasting over two hours. What intervention should be expected?
A. Hydration, pain control, and urologic consultation
B. Application of cold packs and bed rest
C. Foley catheter insertion
D. Initiation of antibiotics

Q481. After receiving asparaginase, a child complains of severe abdominal pain and nausea. Amylase levels are elevated. What does this finding indicate?
A. Nephritis
B. Hepatitis
C. Pancreatitis
D. Cholecystitis

Q482. A child with lymphoma develops facial swelling, distended neck veins, and stridor. What is the nurse's priority action?
A. Elevate the head of the bed
B. Apply a cervical collar
C. Encourage oral hydration
D. Administer antihypertensive medications

Q483. A child undergoing chemotherapy reports sharp pain at the IV site, followed by swelling and redness. What is the nurse's immediate action?
A. Stop the infusion
B. Apply heat to the area
C. Increase the IV rate
D. Flush the site with saline
Q484. A patient with leukemia presents with confusion and seizures after CAR-T cell therapy. What should the nurse do first?
A. Encourage fluid intake
B. Administer broad-spectrum antibiotics
C. Give diuretics
D. Implement seizure precautions and assess airway
Q485. A child with sickle cell anemia has sudden severe pain in long bones and fever. Which nursing action is most appropriate?
A. Begin IV fluids and administer analgesics
B. Apply ice packs to affected area
C. Encourage increased activity
D. Restrict fluids until fever subsides
Q486. A child is receiving chemotherapy becomes suddenly dyspneic with cyanosis and diminished breath sounds on one side. What should the nurse do first?
A. Encourage deep breathing and coughing
B. Call a rapid response and prepare for chest tube insertion
C. Increase IV fluids
D. Position the child supine
Q487. A child treated for neuroblastoma develops profound hypertension and sweating during tumor manipulation. What is the likely cause?
A. Catecholamine release
B. Hemorrhage
C. Dehydration
D. Cardiac tamponade
Q488. A child on high-dose methotrexate therapy develops confusion and elevated creatinine levels. What should the nurse expect to administer?
A. Calcium supplements
B. Allopurinol
C. Leucovorin rescue therapy
D. Insulin infusion
Q489. A child with hemophilia develops knee swelling after a minor fall. Which action should the nurse take first?
A. Administer factor replacement
B. Apply warm compresses
C. Encourage ambulation
D. Elevate the leg after one hour
Q490. A child with leukemia develops increased ICP and vomiting during a platelet transfusion. What is the nurse's immediate response?
A. Stop transfusion and notify provider
B. Continue infusion and assess pain
C. Elevate the foot of the bed
D. Offer oral fluids
Q491. A child receiving chemotherapy becomes suddenly dyspneic with cyanosis and diminished breath sounds on one side. What should the nurse do first?
A. Encourage deep breathing and coughing
B. Call a rapid response and prepare for chest tube insertion
C. Increase IV fluids
D. Position the child supine
Q492. A patient with leukemia has a platelet count of 8,000/mm^3 and develops petechiae. What is the nurse's priority action?
A. Prepare to administer platelet transfusion
B. Encourage physical activity
C. Obtain a urinalysis
D. Begin iron supplementation
Q493. A child receiving asparaginase complains of severe abdominal pain and vomiting. Serum amylase levels are elevated. What complication does the nurse suspect?
A. Pancreatitis
B. Appendicitis
C. Hepatitis
D. Gastroenteritis
Q494. A patient with sickle cell disease presents with fever, hypoxia, and chest pain. What nursing action is most urgent?
A. Encourage oral fluids only
B. Begin corticosteroids
C. Provide antiemetic medication
D. Administer oxygen and antibiotics
Q495. During chemotherapy infusion, a patient develops itching, flushing, and hypotension. What is the nurse's initial response?

A. Stop the infusion and assess airway
B. Increase infusion rate to finish faster
C. Administer saline flush through line
D. Notify provider after medication is completed

Q496. A child with leukemia reports severe headache and blurred vision. Vital signs show hypertension. What is the nurse's priority?

A. Assess for neurologic changes and notify provider
B. Restrict fluids immediately
C. Administer diuretics
D. Provide warm compresses to head

Q497. A patient with neuroblastoma experiences extreme hypertension during tumor manipulation. What intervention should the nurse anticipate?

A. Apply warm blankets
B. Start IV fluids
C. Administration of alpha-adrenergic blockers
D. Administer insulin

Q498. A child with sickle cell anemia reports sudden pallor and weakness. Spleen is enlarged on examination. Which action should the nurse perform first?

A. Prepare for immediate blood transfusion
B. Administer corticosteroids
C. Encourage ambulation
D. Apply heat to the abdomen

Q499. A child receiving ifosfamide develops confusion and seizures. Which medication should the nurse anticipate administering?

A. Dexamethasone
B. Leucovorin
C. Vitamin K
D. Methylene blue

Q500. A patient on total parenteral nutrition after tumor resection has abdominal distension, vomiting, and absent bowel sounds. What complication does the nurse suspect?

A. Bowel obstruction
B. Pancreatitis
C. Peptic ulcer
D. Gastroenteritis

Answer Key and Explanation (401-500)

Q401. Answer: A
Explanation: Ifosfamide can cause encephalopathy from its neurotoxic metabolites, presenting with confusion, hallucinations, or seizures. Stopping the infusion and notifying the provider ensures prompt treatment with methylene blue if indicated. Close monitoring prevents complications.
Subdomain: Neurologic Symptom Management – Chemotherapy Neurotoxicity
Q402. Answer: B
Explanation: Anticipatory nausea is a conditioned response to previous treatment experiences. Combining pharmacologic and behavioral strategies, such as relaxation or guided imagery, minimizes symptoms. Consistency in antiemetic timing improves control.
Subdomain: Gastrointestinal Symptom Management – Anticipatory Nausea
Q403. Answer: A
Explanation: Frequent saline rinses and gentle oral care reduce bacterial colonization and promote healing in mucositis. Alcohol and acidic products worsen irritation. Maintaining hygiene prevents secondary infection.
Subdomain: Oral Mucositis Management
Q404. Answer: A
Explanation: Corticosteroids cause Cushingoid features and mood fluctuations due to metabolic and hormonal effects. These symptoms resolve gradually after therapy tapering. Family education supports adherence and emotional coping.
Subdomain: Endocrine and Metabolic Symptom Management
Q405. Answer: D
Explanation: Peripheral neuropathy affects motor and sensory function, increasing fall and injury risk. Assessing strength and coordination ensures safety and helps determine need for treatment modification.
Subdomain: Neuropathy and Safety Management
Q406. Answer: A
Explanation: Sudden respiratory distress during TPN infusion may indicate air embolism from central line compromise. The nurse should stop infusion, place the patient in left Trendelenburg position, and notify the provider. Prompt action prevents cardiovascular collapse.
Subdomain: Central Line Complication Management
Q407. Answer: A
Explanation: Fatigue and pallor are hallmark signs of anemia caused by chemotherapy-induced bone marrow suppression. Monitoring hemoglobin guides transfusion or dose adjustment. Supportive care includes rest and nutritional support.
Subdomain: Hematologic Symptom Management – Anemia
Q408. Answer: C
Explanation: Radiation-induced mucositis requires soft, nonirritating foods and frequent rinses to maintain comfort and nutrition. Acidic foods worsen irritation. Analgesics before meals promote adequate intake.
Subdomain: Gastrointestinal Symptom Management – Esophagitis
Q409. Answer: A
Explanation: High-dose cytarabine can cause cerebellar toxicity with neurologic symptoms like ataxia and confusion. Immediate cessation and provider notification are essential to prevent permanent damage.
Subdomain: Neurologic Symptom Management – Chemotherapy Neurotoxicity
Q410. Answer: A
Explanation: Elevated liver enzymes indicate hepatotoxicity, a potential side effect of certain chemotherapeutic agents. Holding treatment and notifying the provider prevents progression to hepatic failure. Monitoring bilirubin and AST/ALT guides decisions.
Subdomain: Hepatic Symptom Management
Q411. Answer: D
Explanation: Fever and chills during biotherapy often indicate a cytokine-mediated infusion reaction. Stopping the infusion and assessing the patient ensures stability. Supportive therapy can be initiated once symptoms resolve.

Subdomain: Biotherapy – Infusion Reaction Management

Q412. Answer: A

Explanation: Cyclophosphamide's metabolite acrolein can irritate the bladder, causing hemorrhagic cystitis. Aggressive hydration and frequent voiding help eliminate the irritant. Mesna provides additional bladder protection.

Subdomain: Urologic Symptom Management

Q413. Answer: A

Explanation: Gentle moisturizing protects irradiated skin and promotes healing. Alcohol and friction worsen irritation. Teaching includes avoiding sunlight and using loose, soft fabrics.

Subdomain: Integumentary Symptom Management – Radiation Dermatitis

Q414. Answer: C

Explanation: Social withdrawal is common due to fatigue, anxiety, and body image changes during therapy. Encouraging age-appropriate engagement fosters psychosocial well-being and resilience. Support from peers reduces isolation.

Subdomain: Psychosocial Symptom Management

Q415. Answer: A

Explanation: Sinusoidal obstruction syndrome results from hepatic venule injury following conditioning regimens. Symptoms include hepatomegaly, ascites, and jaundice. Supportive management includes fluid restriction and defibrotide therapy.

Subdomain: Hepatic and Metabolic Symptom Management

Q416. Answer: A

Explanation: Thrombocytopenia increases bleeding risk. Teaching includes avoiding trauma, using soft toothbrushes, and not using aspirin or NSAIDs. Early recognition of bleeding signs ensures timely intervention.

Subdomain: Hematologic Symptom Management – Bleeding Risk

Q417. Answer: B

Explanation: Chemotherapy damages oral mucosa, leading to painful ulcerations and bleeding. Gentle saline rinses and topical anesthetics relieve discomfort and prevent infection. Soft oral care tools are essential for mucosal integrity.

Subdomain: Oral and Mucosal Care

Q418. Answer: A

Explanation: Vincristine-induced peripheral neuropathy may progress to motor weakness or foot drop. Immediate assessment and reporting prevent permanent damage. Dose adjustments are often required to protect function.

Subdomain: Neuropathy Management – Motor Impairment

Q419. Answer: A

Explanation: Respiratory depression from opioid toxicity is life-threatening. Naloxone administration reverses the effects rapidly and restores ventilation. Close monitoring prevents recurrence after reversal.

Subdomain: Pain Management – Opioid Overdose

Q420. Answer: C

Explanation: Tumor lysis syndrome results from rapid tumor cell destruction, causing hyperkalemia, hyperphosphatemia, and hypocalcemia. Symptoms include cramps, confusion, and arrhythmias. Prompt hydration and allopurinol or rasburicase prevent renal failure.

Subdomain: Metabolic Emergency Management – Tumor Lysis Syndrome

Q421. Answer: A

Explanation: Methotrexate can crystallize in renal tubules, causing nephrotoxicity and oliguria. Adequate hydration and urine alkalinization prevent toxicity. Immediate provider notification ensures leucovorin adjustment and renal protection.

Subdomain: Renal Symptom Management – Chemotherapy Nephrotoxicity

Q422. Answer: A

Explanation: Immunocompromised children are at high risk for opportunistic infections such as Pneumocystis jirovecii. Symptoms include fever, dry cough, and respiratory distress. Prophylaxis with trimethoprim-sulfamethoxazole and early detection improve outcomes.

Subdomain: Pulmonary Symptom Management – Opportunistic Infections

Q423. Answer: B

Explanation: These are signs of a severe cytokine release reaction, a medical emergency during

biotherapy. Stopping infusion and initiating emergency protocols, including fluids and possible tocilizumab, are life-saving measures.
Subdomain: Biotherapy Symptom Management – Cytokine Release Syndrome

Q424. Answer: A

Explanation: Thick saliva and dysphagia result from radiation-induced glandular damage. Frequent water intake and bland rinses maintain comfort and oral hygiene. Avoiding acidic or dry foods prevents further irritation.
Subdomain: Oral and Gastrointestinal Symptom Management – Xerostomia

Q425. Answer: A

Explanation: Vincristine-induced neuropathy slows gastrointestinal motility, leading to constipation and bloating. Early bowel regimens prevent ileus and discomfort. Adequate hydration and dietary fiber further promote bowel regularity.
Subdomain: Gastrointestinal Symptom Management – Constipation

Q426. Answer: D

Explanation: Opioid-induced nausea occurs due to stimulation of the chemoreceptor trigger zone. Administering antiemetics before and after dosing enhances comfort and allows continued pain control. Monitoring response ensures balance between relief and side effects.
Subdomain: Pain Management – Opioid Side Effects

Q427. Answer: A

Explanation: Anthracyclines such as doxorubicin may cause cumulative cardiomyopathy. Symptoms like dyspnea or fatigue warrant echocardiographic evaluation. Early detection helps adjust treatment and prevent cardiac failure.
Subdomain: Cardiovascular Symptom Management – Anthracycline Toxicity

Q428. Answer: A

Explanation: Acute graft-versus-host disease (GVHD) results from donor T-cell attack on host tissues, typically skin, liver, and gut. Rash, diarrhea, and jaundice are characteristic findings. Prompt immunosuppressive therapy prevents severe organ damage.
Subdomain: Immune-Related Complication Management

Q429. Answer: B

Explanation: Peripheral neuropathy affects fine motor skills and increases injury risk. Comprehensive assessment allows appropriate precautions and potential treatment adjustments. Safety and functional independence remain primary nursing goals.
Subdomain: Neuropathy Management – Functional Assessment

Q430. Answer: A

Explanation: Thrombocytopenia increases bleeding risk; avoiding trauma and invasive procedures is essential. Soft oral care and activity modification prevent further bleeding. Monitoring platelet count guides supportive transfusions.
Subdomain: Hematologic Symptom Management – Bleeding Precautions

Q431. Answer: A

Explanation: Rapid IV fluid resuscitation is critical to maintain perfusion and prevent progression to septic shock. Children often require repeated isotonic boluses before vasopressor support. Delays in fluid administration significantly worsen outcomes.
Subdomain: Infection – Sepsis

Q432. Answer: C

Explanation: Typhlitis is a life-threatening bowel inflammation in neutropenic patients. The nurse must stop oral intake to reduce risk of perforation and immediately notify the provider for imaging and IV antibiotics. Early bowel rest prevents complications.
Subdomain: Infection – Typhlitis

Q433. Answer: A

Explanation: Tumor lysis syndrome causes rapid electrolyte shifts and uric acid accumulation. Vigorous IV hydration promotes renal clearance, and allopurinol or rasburicase reduces uric acid formation. Prompt management prevents renal failure.
Subdomain: Metabolic – Tumor Lysis Syndrome

Q434. Answer: A

Explanation: Disseminated intravascular coagulation consumes clotting factors, leading to bleeding. Replacement with plasma and

cryoprecipitate replenishes fibrinogen and clotting proteins. Continuous monitoring for bleeding is essential during therapy.
Subdomain: Vascular – Disseminated Intravascular Coagulation

Q435. Answer: B

Explanation: Positional dyspnea suggests compression of the superior vena cava by the mass. Elevating the head facilitates venous return and reduces airway obstruction until definitive therapy begins. This position minimizes respiratory distress.
Subdomain: Cardiopulmonary – Superior Vena Cava Syndrome

Q436. Answer: A

Explanation: Elevation of the head promotes venous drainage and lowers intracranial pressure. Trendelenburg and Valsalva maneuvers can worsen pressure and increase risk for herniation. Neurologic assessment should be performed frequently.
Subdomain: Neurology – Increased Intracranial Pressure

Q437. Answer: A

Explanation: Syndrome of inappropriate antidiuretic hormone secretion causes water retention and hyponatremia. Controlled fluid restriction corrects dilutional sodium imbalance. Monitoring weight and serum sodium guides safe management.
Subdomain: Metabolic – SIADH

Q438. Answer: D

Explanation: Acute chest syndrome occurs when sickled cells obstruct pulmonary vasculature, causing hypoxia and pain. It requires immediate oxygen, antibiotics, and transfusion support. Delay can rapidly lead to respiratory failure.
Subdomain: Cardiopulmonary – Acute Chest Syndrome

Q439. Answer: A

Explanation: Posterior reversible encephalopathy syndrome is linked to hypertension or immunosuppressive drugs like cyclosporine. It presents with seizures, headache, and visual changes. Management includes blood pressure control and drug adjustment.
Subdomain: Neurology – PRES

Q440. Answer: A

Explanation: Splenic sequestration causes pooling of blood within the spleen, leading to hypovolemia and shock. Prompt transfusion restores circulating volume and oxygen delivery. Delayed intervention can be fatal.
Subdomain: Vascular – Splenic Sequestration

Q441. Answer: C

Explanation: Sinusoidal obstructive syndrome, or veno-occlusive disease, causes hepatic congestion and jaundice following conditioning therapy. Early recognition and supportive fluid management reduce risk of hepatic failure.
Subdomain: Vascular – Sinusoidal Obstructive Syndrome

Q442. Answer: A

Explanation: Joint bleeds require prompt immobilization and cold application to limit bleeding. Factor replacement follows to stop the hemorrhage. Early care prevents chronic arthropathy.
Subdomain: Vascular – Joint Bleed (Hemophilia)

Q443. Answer: A

Explanation: Neuroblastomas can release catecholamines during surgery, causing hypertensive crises. Blood pressure must be monitored closely, and alpha-blockade may be needed for control. Immediate recognition prevents cardiac complications.
Subdomain: Metabolic – Catecholamine Excess

Q444. Answer: B

Explanation: Anaphylaxis requires stopping the medication and ensuring airway support. Epinephrine and emergency interventions should follow per protocol. Delaying response can result in respiratory collapse.
Subdomain: Hypersensitivity Reactions

Q445. Answer: A

Explanation: Extravasation of vesicant drugs causes tissue necrosis. Stopping the infusion prevents further damage, and antidotes or cold compresses may be applied depending on the agent. Prompt reporting ensures rapid management.
Subdomain: Extravasation

Q446. Answer: A

Explanation: Methotrexate toxicity is worsened by acidic urine and poor clearance. Maintaining

alkalinized urine and timely leucovorin rescue prevent renal and neurological complications. Monitoring labs ensures early detection.
Subdomain: Metabolic – Drug-Induced Toxicity

Q447. Answer: C

Explanation: Vaso-occlusive crisis results from sickled cells obstructing blood flow. Assessing hydration and oxygen supports targeted interventions that restore perfusion. Adequate fluids and oxygen reduce further sickling.
Subdomain: Vascular – Vaso-occlusive Crisis

Q448. Answer: A

Explanation: Graft-versus-host disease occurs when donor immune cells attack host tissues, commonly skin, liver, and GI tract. Prompt immunosuppressive therapy is vital to limit damage. Early signs require immediate reporting.
Subdomain: Immune – Graft-versus-Host Response

Q449. Answer: A

Explanation: Cytokine release syndrome is a severe inflammatory response following CAR-T therapy. Early recognition and administration of tocilizumab or corticosteroids can prevent multi-organ failure. Close monitoring in ICU is often needed.
Subdomain: Metabolic – Cytokine Release Syndrome

Q450. Answer: B

Explanation: Bowel obstruction may result from tumor recurrence or postoperative adhesions. Symptoms include distension, vomiting, and absent bowel sounds. Early nasogastric decompression and imaging are indicated.
Subdomain: Gastrointestinal – Bowel Obstruction

Q451. Answer: C

Explanation: Fluid resuscitation is vital to restore perfusion during septic shock in immunocompromised children. Early aggressive isotonic fluids improve cardiac output and prevent organ failure. Timing of fluids significantly influences survival.
Subdomain: Infection – Sepsis

Q452. Answer: C

Explanation: These symptoms may indicate neutropenic enterocolitis, a surgical emergency. The nurse should stop oral intake and inform the provider immediately. IV antibiotics and bowel rest are required to prevent perforation.
Subdomain: Infection – Typhlitis

Q453. Answer: B

Explanation: Oxygen saturation below 90% indicates severe respiratory compromise. This may signal pneumonia or acute chest syndrome in immunocompromised patients. Immediate oxygen therapy and provider notification are essential.
Subdomain: Infection – Pulmonary Complication

Q454. Answer: C

Explanation: Transfusion reactions require immediate discontinuation of the infusion to prevent anaphylaxis or hemolysis. The nurse should maintain IV access with saline and report findings promptly. Documentation of reaction details is crucial.
Subdomain: Hypersensitivity – Transfusion Reaction

Q455. Answer: A

Explanation: A pH below 7.35 indicates acidosis. Chemotherapy-related lactic acidosis can occur from tissue hypoxia or hepatic impairment. Identifying and treating the cause early prevents cardiovascular collapse.
Subdomain: Metabolic – Acidosis

Q456. Answer: A

Explanation: Tocilizumab, an interleukin-6 receptor blocker, mitigates inflammatory cytokine effects during cytokine release syndrome. Early intervention prevents multiorgan dysfunction. Monitoring for rapid deterioration is crucial.
Subdomain: Metabolic – Cytokine Release Syndrome

Q457. Answer: A

Explanation: Persistent hypotension after fluid resuscitation indicates septic shock requiring vasopressor support. Dopamine or norepinephrine helps maintain perfusion until the infection is controlled. Continuous monitoring is mandatory.
Subdomain: Infection – Septic Shock

Q458. Answer: B

Explanation: Splenic sequestration causes blood pooling and hypovolemia. Rapid transfusion

restores circulating volume and prevents cardiovascular collapse. Pain management follows stabilization.
Subdomain: Vascular – Splenic Sequestration

Q459. Answer: A

Explanation: Vincristine may cause peripheral neuropathy, leading to muscle weakness or gait disturbances. Early provider notification allows dose modification to prevent permanent damage. Regular neuromuscular assessments are essential.
Subdomain: Neurology – Drug-Induced Neuropathy

Q460. Answer: A

Explanation: Acute chest syndrome is treated urgently with oxygen to correct hypoxia and antibiotics to address possible infection. Early recognition and transfusion may prevent respiratory failure.
Subdomain: Cardiopulmonary – Acute Chest Syndrome

Q461. Answer: D

Explanation: Cytokine-related neurotoxicity can cause seizures and cerebral edema. Airway protection and seizure precautions are immediate priorities. The provider should be notified for further management and medication orders.
Subdomain: Neurology – Immune Effector Cell–Associated Neurotoxicity

Q462. Answer: A

Explanation: Certain agents, such as cyclophosphamide, can cause bladder mucosal irritation leading to hemorrhagic cystitis. Hydration and mesna are used for prevention. Prompt reporting prevents renal compromise.
Subdomain: Genitourinary – Hemorrhagic Cystitis

Q463. Answer: A

Explanation: Hyperleukocytosis can cause cerebrovascular congestion and neurological symptoms. Leukapheresis rapidly reduces circulating blasts, preventing stroke and respiratory distress. Immediate intervention is life-saving.
Subdomain: Vascular – Hyperleukocytosis

Q464. Answer: C

Explanation: Adequate hydration and oxygen reduce sickling and restore blood flow. Pain management is essential but should accompany physiologic interventions that address the crisis cause.
Subdomain: Vascular – Vaso-occlusive Crisis

Q465. Answer: A

Explanation: Sinusoidal obstructive syndrome is caused by hepatic venous occlusion following conditioning regimens. Supportive care and fluid balance monitoring are essential to prevent liver failure.
Subdomain: Vascular – Sinusoidal Obstructive Syndrome

Q466. Answer: A

Explanation: Papilledema indicates increased intracranial pressure due to CNS infiltration or hydrocephalus. Immediate intervention prevents brain herniation. The nurse should notify the provider promptly.
Subdomain: Neurology – Increased Intracranial Pressure

Q467. Answer: B

Explanation: Tumor lysis releases intracellular phosphate, binding calcium and lowering serum levels. Resulting hypocalcemia causes tetany and confusion. Early hydration and medication reduce severity.
Subdomain: Metabolic – Tumor Lysis Syndrome

Q468. Answer: A

Explanation: Steroids and asparaginase can trigger pancreatitis in pediatric oncology patients. Prompt withholding of the offending drug and supportive therapy are key to prevent necrosis.
Subdomain: Gastrointestinal – Pancreatitis

Q469. Answer: A

Explanation: Cardiac arrest requires immediate CPR to restore circulation and oxygenation. Defibrillation and emergency medications follow per protocol. Quick recognition and action determine survival.
Subdomain: Cardiopulmonary – Cardiac Arrest

Q470. Answer: C

Explanation: Ifosfamide can cross the blood–brain barrier and cause neurotoxicity presenting as confusion or seizures. Discontinuation of the

drug and methylene blue therapy are typical treatments.
Subdomain: Neurology – Drug-Induced Encephalopathy

Q471. Answer: B

Explanation: Tumor lysis syndrome can cause life-threatening hyperkalemia and acute renal failure. Dialysis or continuous renal replacement therapy may be necessary when medical management fails. Prompt escalation prevents cardiac arrest.
Subdomain: Metabolic – Tumor Lysis Syndrome

Q472. Answer: A

Explanation: Oxygen therapy is the first priority to correct hypoxia in acute chest syndrome. Early antibiotic administration and transfusion follow once the condition is stabilized. This approach prevents respiratory failure.
Subdomain: Cardiopulmonary – Acute Chest Syndrome

Q473. Answer: C

Explanation: Cyclophosphamide metabolites irritate the bladder and cause hemorrhagic cystitis. Increasing hydration helps flush toxic metabolites and prevents permanent bladder injury. Mesna may be prescribed as a protective agent.
Subdomain: Genitourinary – Hemorrhagic Cystitis

Q474. Answer: A

Explanation: Sinusoidal obstructive syndrome (veno-occlusive disease) results from hepatic venule blockage. Defibrotide improves hepatic microcirculation and reduces mortality. Fluid restriction and daily weights are key supportive measures.
Subdomain: Vascular – Sinusoidal Obstructive Syndrome

Q475. Answer: D

Explanation: Acute hypersensitivity reactions require immediate discontinuation of the infusion to prevent anaphylaxis. Airway maintenance is critical while emergency medications are prepared. Documentation follows stabilization.
Subdomain: Hypersensitivity Reaction

Q476. Answer: A

Explanation: Splenic sequestration leads to sudden pooling of blood in the spleen, causing hypovolemic shock. Immediate transfusion restores blood volume and oxygen-carrying capacity. Continuous monitoring is essential for stability.
Subdomain: Vascular – Splenic Sequestration

Q477. Answer: A

Explanation: Cytarabine can cause cerebellar toxicity, manifesting as confusion, ataxia, and slurred speech. Early recognition and drug suspension prevent irreversible neurological damage. Neurologic checks should be performed before each dose.
Subdomain: Neurology – Drug-Induced Neurotoxicity

Q478. Answer: D

Explanation: Unilateral breath sound loss following line placement suggests pneumothorax. Immediate provider notification and preparation for needle decompression or chest tube insertion are critical to reestablish ventilation.
Subdomain: Cardiopulmonary – Respiratory Distress

Q479. Answer: A

Explanation: Extreme leukocytosis can lead to blood viscosity and cerebrovascular obstruction, increasing stroke risk. Rapid leukapheresis or exchange transfusion helps prevent complications. Continuous neuro checks are warranted.
Subdomain: Vascular – Hyperleukocytosis

Q480. Answer: A

Explanation: Prolonged priapism results from vaso-occlusion and can cause permanent erectile dysfunction. Hydration and pain control relieve ischemia, while urology intervention ensures decompression if needed.
Subdomain: Vascular – Priapism

Q481. Answer: C

Explanation: Asparaginase may cause pancreatic inflammation resulting in elevated amylase and abdominal pain. The medication should be discontinued and the provider notified immediately. Supportive management prevents further injury.
Subdomain: Gastrointestinal – Pancreatitis

Q482. Answer: A

Explanation: Superior vena cava obstruction from mediastinal compression restricts venous return. Elevating the head promotes drainage and eases respiratory distress until corticosteroid or radiation therapy is initiated.

Subdomain: Cardiopulmonary – Superior Vena Cava Syndrome

Q483. Answer: A

Explanation: Extravasation of vesicant chemotherapy can cause severe tissue necrosis. The infusion must be stopped immediately to prevent worsening injury. Depending on the agent, antidotes or cold compresses may be indicated.

Subdomain: Extravasation

Q484. Answer: D

Explanation: Cytokine-related neurotoxicity following CAR-T therapy can rapidly progress to cerebral edema. Ensuring airway patency and seizure safety are immediate priorities. The provider should be alerted for further treatment.

Subdomain: Neurology – CAR-T Neurotoxicity

Q485. Answer: A

Explanation: Vaso-occlusive crisis results from obstruction of blood flow by sickled cells. Hydration improves blood viscosity, and analgesics manage severe pain. Rest and warmth support tissue oxygenation.

Subdomain: Vascular – Vaso-occlusive Crisis

Q486. Answer: A

Explanation: Anaphylaxis presents with hypotension and airway compromise shortly after transfusion. Immediate discontinuation of transfusion and emergency treatment with epinephrine are vital to prevent collapse.

Subdomain: Hypersensitivity – Transfusion Reaction

Q487. Answer: A

Explanation: Neuroblastoma tumors may release catecholamines intraoperatively, causing hypertensive crisis. Continuous blood pressure monitoring and prompt use of alpha-blockers are essential.

Subdomain: Metabolic – Catecholamine Excess

Q488. Answer: C

Explanation: Leucovorin counteracts methotrexate toxicity by rescuing healthy cells. Adequate hydration and alkalinization of urine are essential to enhance methotrexate clearance. Renal monitoring continues throughout therapy.

Subdomain: Metabolic – Drug-Induced Toxicity

Q489. Answer: A

Explanation: Prompt replacement of the deficient clotting factor halts bleeding and prevents joint damage. Immobilization and ice follow to reduce pain and inflammation. Delay in replacement worsens hemarthrosis.

Subdomain: Vascular – Joint Bleed (Hemophilia)

Q490. Answer: A

Explanation: Neurological changes during transfusion may signal intracranial bleeding or acute reaction. Stopping the transfusion prevents further complications while the cause is investigated. Neurologic assessment must follow urgently.

Subdomain: Neurology – Transfusion-Related Complication

Q491. Answer: B

Explanation: Unilateral breath sound loss and cyanosis suggest a pneumothorax, often caused by line placement or tumor involvement. Immediate provider notification and preparation for chest decompression are vital to restore oxygenation.

Subdomain: Cardiopulmonary – Pneumothorax

Q492. Answer: A

Explanation: A platelet count below $10{,}000/mm^3$ places the patient at high risk for spontaneous bleeding. Prompt transfusion replenishes clotting elements and prevents hemorrhage. Bleeding precautions must be enforced immediately.

Subdomain: Hematologic – Thrombocytopenia

Q493. Answer: A

Explanation: Asparaginase can inflame the pancreas, leading to acute pancreatitis. Immediate discontinuation of the drug and supportive care reduce the risk of necrosis or infection. The provider should be notified promptly.

Subdomain: Gastrointestinal – Pancreatitis

Q494. Answer: D

Explanation: Acute chest syndrome requires prompt oxygenation to relieve hypoxia and

antibiotics to treat underlying infection. Supportive care including pain control and transfusion may be required to prevent respiratory failure.
Subdomain: Cardiopulmonary – Acute Chest Syndrome

Q495. Answer: A

Explanation: These signs indicate a hypersensitivity reaction. Stopping the infusion prevents further exposure while airway and hemodynamic stability are assessed. Emergency medications such as epinephrine may be required.
Subdomain: Hypersensitivity Reaction

Q496. Answer: A

Explanation: Headache and visual disturbances with elevated blood pressure may indicate increased intracranial pressure or posterior reversible encephalopathy. Early neurologic assessment and provider notification prevent irreversible damage.
Subdomain: Neurology – Increased Intracranial Pressure

Q497. Answer: C

Explanation: Catecholamine-secreting tumors can cause hypertensive crises. Alpha-blockers such as phenoxybenzamine stabilize blood pressure before or during surgery. Continuous monitoring prevents life-threatening complications.
Subdomain: Metabolic – Catecholamine Excess

Q498. Answer: A

Explanation: Splenic sequestration crisis results in hypovolemia and rapid decline in hemoglobin. Blood transfusion restores circulating volume and oxygenation. Monitoring for shock is essential throughout management.
Subdomain: Vascular – Splenic Sequestration

Q499. Answer: D

Explanation: Ifosfamide-induced encephalopathy is treated with methylene blue, which reverses neurotoxic metabolites. Discontinuation of the offending agent and supportive measures help recovery. Continuous neuro checks are essential.
Subdomain: Neurology – Drug-Induced Encephalopathy

Q500. Answer: A

Explanation: Bowel obstruction presents with distension and vomiting due to impaired intestinal flow. Early detection and nasogastric decompression prevent perforation and shock. The nurse should notify the provider immediately.
Subdomain: Gastrointestinal – Bowel Obstruction

Question (501-600)

Q501. A child develops dyspnea, tachycardia, and chest tightness shortly after blood transfusion. What should the nurse do first?

A. Stop the transfusion and keep IV line open with saline
B. Administer analgesics for chest discomfort
C. Check temperature and resume transfusion
D. Encourage coughing and deep breathing

Q502. After high-dose chemotherapy, a child presents with elevated uric acid and potassium levels. Which preventive measure is most appropriate?

A. Restricting fluid intake
B. Vigorous IV hydration
C. Administering iron supplements
D. Encouraging high-protein diet

Q503. A child with sickle cell disease reports priapism lasting over two hours. What nursing intervention should the nurse implement first?

A. Encourage hydration and administer pain medication
B. Apply cold compresses
C. Restrict fluids until episode resolves
D. Encourage ambulation

Q504. A child undergoing CAR-T therapy develops fever, hypotension, and tachypnea. What immediate treatment does the nurse anticipate?

A. Tocilizumab
B. Vancomycin
C. Epinephrine
D. Albumin infusion

Q505. A patient with sickle cell disease presents with leg pain unrelieved by acetaminophen. What is the next nursing action?

A. Apply cold packs
B. Encourage ambulation
C. Administer IV fluids and opioid analgesics
D. Restrict fluids

Q506. A child with leukemia develops fever, tachycardia, and capillary refill >3 seconds. Despite fluids, hypotension persists. What should the nurse anticipate?

A. Initiation of vasopressor support
B. Discontinuing fluids
C. Starting blood transfusion
D. Restricting sodium intake

Q507. A child on vincristine reports numbness in hands and difficulty buttoning clothes. What is the best nursing action?

A. Report symptoms for possible dose adjustment
B. Encourage fine motor exercises
C. Apply compression gloves
D. Continue therapy as ordered

Q508. After hematopoietic stem cell transplant, a patient presents with watery diarrhea, rash, and jaundice. What condition should the nurse suspect?

A. Drug toxicity
B. Sepsis
C. Allergic dermatitis
D. Graft-versus-host disease

Q509. A child receiving daunorubicin reports new onset of shortness of breath and fatigue. Which finding would confirm the suspected complication?

A. Decreased ejection fraction on echocardiogram
B. Elevated white blood cell count
C. Increased liver enzymes
D. Hypocalcemia

Q510. A patient receiving chemotherapy presents with severe nausea, headache, and seizures. Serum sodium is 118 mEq/L. What intervention should the nurse anticipate?

A. Fluid restriction and hypertonic saline administration
B. Increase oral fluid intake
C. Encourage diuretics
D. Administer potassium supplements

Q511. A child receiving induction chemotherapy presents with severe vomiting, confusion, and muscle twitching. Serum calcium is 6.5 mg/dL, and phosphorus is elevated. What is the most likely cause?

A. Syndrome of inappropriate antidiuretic hormone
B. Tumor lysis syndrome
C. Diabetes insipidus
D. Hepatic failure

Q512. A child receiving ifosfamide suddenly becomes disoriented and unable to follow

commands. What medication does the nurse anticipate administering?
A. Leucovorin
B. Methylene blue
C. Allopurinol
D. Corticosteroid
Q513. A child post-transplant develops weight gain, right upper quadrant pain, and jaundice. Which nursing action takes priority?
A. Notify provider and prepare to administer defibrotide
B. Encourage high-protein diet
C. Apply warm compresses to abdomen
D. Restrict activity
Q514. A child with sickle cell disease reports back and joint pain unrelieved by acetaminophen. What is the next nursing intervention?
A. Administer IV fluids and opioid analgesics
B. Encourage ambulation
C. Apply ice packs to painful areas
D. Restrict oral fluids
Q515. During a platelet transfusion, a child develops fever, chills, and hypotension. What should the nurse do first?
A. Elevate legs to improve blood flow
B. Give acetaminophen and continue slowly
C. Stop transfusion and maintain IV access with saline
D. Record symptoms after completion
Q516. A child with leukemia reports sudden headache, vomiting, and blurred vision. What complication should the nurse suspect?
A. Increased intracranial pressure
B. Hypoglycemia
C. Hypercalcemia
D. Cerebral embolism
Q517. A patient undergoing CAR-T cell therapy develops high fever and hypotension. Which medication does the nurse anticipate?
A. Tocilizumab
B. Epinephrine
C. Dexamethasone
D. Cefepime
Q518. A child with hemophilia complains of elbow pain and swelling after a fall. What should the nurse do first?
A. Elevate arm after four hours
B. Apply warm compresses
C. Encourage range-of-motion exercises
D. Administer factor replacement
Q519. A child receiving vincristine develops numbness in fingers and toes. Which nursing action is appropriate?
A. Notify provider of potential neuropathy
B. Apply warm packs
C. Encourage fine-motor activities
D. Continue therapy as scheduled
Q520. A child with leukemia develops respiratory distress and jugular vein distention. What is the nurse's immediate action?
A. Elevate head of bed and monitor oxygen saturation
B. Place child supine
C. Start vigorous chest physiotherapy
D. Encourage deep breathing
Q521. After high-dose chemotherapy, a child develops hyponatremia, weight gain, and low urine output. What is the likely cause?
A. Dehydration
B. Diabetes insipidus
C. SIADH
D. Tumor lysis syndrome
Q522. A child with sickle cell disease suddenly develops tachypnea, chest pain, and new infiltrate on chest X-ray. What is the best initial treatment?
A. Oxygen therapy and antibiotics
B. Steroids only
C. Antihistamines and IV fluids
D. Blood culture and wait for results
Q523. A child receiving cyclophosphamide complains of burning during urination and blood in urine. What should the nurse do?
A. Increase IV hydration and notify provider
B. Restrict fluids
C. Apply heat to lower abdomen
D. Encourage caffeine intake
Q524. A child receiving daunorubicin reports fatigue and dyspnea. Which diagnostic test should the nurse expect?
A. Chest X-ray
B. Brain MRI
C. Abdominal ultrasound
D. Echocardiogram

Q525. A child develops severe abdominal pain and elevated lipase during asparaginase therapy. What is the priority action?
A. Stop drug and notify provider
B. Provide antiemetic
C. Administer IV glucose
D. Encourage oral fluids

Q526. A child with leukemia experiences seizures and hypertension. MRI reveals white-matter edema. What condition is indicated?
A. Posterior reversible encephalopathy syndrome
B. Intracranial bleed
C. Hydrocephalus
D. Brain abscess

Q527. A post-transplant patient develops rash, diarrhea, and jaundice two weeks after engraftment. What should the nurse suspect?
A. Hepatitis B infection
B. Graft-versus-host disease
C. Allergic reaction
D. Drug-induced hepatitis

Q528. A child receiving chemotherapy develops blood pressure 80/45 mm Hg after two fluid boluses. Which intervention should the nurse anticipate next?
A. Vasopressor infusion initiation
B. Discontinuing fluids
C. Platelet transfusion
D. Oral electrolyte replacement

Q529. A child with sickle cell disease experiences prolonged penile erection unrelieved by analgesics. What nursing action is appropriate?
A. Notify provider and prepare for aspiration or exchange transfusion
B. Apply ice packs
C. Encourage ambulation
D. Provide sedatives

Q530. A child receiving high-dose methotrexate develops confusion and decreased urine output. Which intervention should be prioritized?
A. Give iron supplements
B. Administer potassium chloride
C. Restrict fluids
D. Verify urine pH and ensure leucovorin rescue

Q531. A 14-year-old with osteosarcoma expresses anger and refuses to participate in physical therapy after an amputation. The nurse's best response is to:
A. Encourage the patient to focus on recovery goals
B. Allow time for emotional expression without judgment
C. Emphasize the importance of rehabilitation
D. Suggest discussing feelings with peers later

Q532. The parents of a 6-year-old newly diagnosed with leukemia alternate between denial and anger. The most appropriate nursing action is to:
A. Provide reassurance that such reactions are normal
B. Offer educational materials on leukemia treatment
C. Encourage them to focus on the positive prognosis
D. Recommend immediate counseling intervention

Q533. A nurse notices that an adolescent patient with sickle cell disease avoids interactions and frequently asks if the pain will ever stop. The most therapeutic response is to:
A. Reassure the patient that pain will improve with time
B. Explore what the pain means to the patient emotionally
C. Distract the patient with activities
D. Emphasize the effectiveness of medication

Q534. During palliative care for a 9-year-old, the nurse observes the parents arguing about treatment decisions. The nurse should first:
A. Arrange a family conference with the care team
B. Suggest postponing decisions until they agree
C. Speak to the physician about conflict mediation
D. Encourage the parents to focus on the child's needs

Q535. A child nearing end of life asks if dying will hurt. The nurse's most appropriate response is to:
A. Divert the conversation to positive memories
B. Explain honestly that comfort measures will prevent pain

C. Ask why the child is thinking about death
D. Reassure that dying is peaceful

Q536. A 12-year-old with lymphoma tells the nurse, "My friends stopped visiting because they think I'm contagious." The nurse should:
A. Explain that this happens often during treatment
B. Offer to talk to the school nurse about peer education
C. Encourage the patient to ignore the situation
D. Suggest joining an online support group only

Q537. Parents of a 3-year-old newly diagnosed with neuroblastoma express guilt, believing they caused the illness. The nurse's best action is to:
A. Provide reassurance that no one is to blame
B. Encourage them to focus on the treatment plan
C. Redirect them toward hopeful outcomes
D. Involve a social worker immediately

Q538. A teenager receiving long-term chemotherapy feels isolated from friends and expresses a loss of identity. The nurse's best intervention is to:
A. Encourage journaling and peer support group participation
B. Provide distraction through hospital activities
C. Arrange for more frequent family visits
D. Increase schoolwork to maintain normalcy

Q539. A family from a different cultural background insists on using herbal remedies alongside chemotherapy. The nurse's best initial step is to:
A. Replace herbs with prescribed vitamins
B. Explain the potential risks and refuse permission
C. Inform the oncologist immediately
D. Respectfully explore their beliefs and practices

Q540. During discharge teaching, a nurse notices that the caregiver of a child with sickle cell disease appears withdrawn and tearful. The most appropriate action is to:
A. Provide emotional support and assess coping needs
B. Focus on reviewing medication instructions
C. Suggest joining a community resource group later
D. Continue the session without interruption

Q541. A nurse caring for an adolescent with relapsed leukemia notices the patient refusing medications and expressing hopelessness. The priority action is to:
A. Assess for depression and suicidal ideation
B. Reinforce the need for treatment adherence
C. Notify parents about the behavior
D. Arrange for distraction therapy

Q542. A 5-year-old undergoing radiation therapy refuses to eat, saying "food tastes bad." The nurse can best assist by:
A. Using rewards for finishing meals
B. Explaining the need for nutrition to recover
C. Offering small, appealing meals and family mealtime support
D. Requesting a feeding tube placement

Q543. The mother of a child with aplastic anemia reports constant fatigue from caregiving. The nurse's best recommendation is to:
A. Utilize respite care or community volunteer programs
B. Focus on time management strategies
C. Take rest when the child naps
D. Seek counseling for anxiety

Q544. A school-age child expresses fear about returning to class due to hair loss. The nurse's best response is to:
A. Offer options like hats or scarves for confidence
B. Tell the child classmates will understand
C. Suggest avoiding school until hair regrows
D. Advise the teacher to minimize attention to it

Q545. After the death of a child, the nurse plans a follow-up call to the family. The primary goal is to:
A. Discuss the child's medical care
B. Evaluate family coping mechanisms
C. Encourage them to return to routines quickly
D. Offer emotional support and provide bereavement resources

Q546. A nurse notes that parents of a child with hemophilia disagree on who should administer factor infusions at home. The best nursing action is to:
A. Facilitate a family teaching session for shared competence

B. Assign one parent as the primary caregiver
C. Notify the physician of disagreement
D. Delay home care training until resolved

Q547. An adolescent with bone marrow failure expresses frustration about missing sports and social events. The most supportive nursing intervention is to:
A. Explore alternative hobbies and virtual connections
B. Emphasize adherence to activity restrictions
C. Remind the patient that health is the priority
D. Encourage focusing on academic success instead

Q548. A nurse caring for a child with chronic anemia observes that siblings feel neglected. The best intervention is to:
A. Arrange for extended family to assist with care
B. Recommend counseling for the siblings
C. Include siblings in age-appropriate discussions and care
D. Provide separate activities to distract them

Q549. During hospitalization, a 7-year-old refuses medication unless a parent gives it. The nurse's best strategy is to:
A. Encourage parent participation during administration
B. Enforce independence by having staff administer it
C. Delay medication until the child complies
D. Use distraction techniques only

Q550. A parent of a terminally ill child expresses guilt for wanting the child's suffering to end. The nurse's most therapeutic response is to:
A. Acknowledge the difficulty and normalize the emotion
B. Redirect to focus on cherished memories
C. Encourage optimism about treatment
D. Avoid discussing emotional conflict

Q551. A 7-year-old with acute lymphoblastic leukemia asks the nurse, "Am I going to die like the other kid in my room?" The nurse's best response is to:
A. Change the subject to something positive
B. Say that everyone's illness is different and ask what the child knows about death
C. Reassure that the doctors will make them better
D. Tell the parents to handle the discussion later

Q552. The parents of a 4-year-old with neuroblastoma express frustration with frequent hospitalizations. The nurse's best intervention is to:
A. Encourage them to focus on the child's progress
B. Offer emotional validation and discuss community support options
C. Remind them that treatment interruptions are harmful
D. Advise scheduling fewer hospital visits

Q553. An adolescent with hemophilia refuses to wear a medical alert bracelet, stating it makes them "look different." The nurse should:
A. Suggest customizing the bracelet to fit personal style
B. Emphasize that the bracelet is mandatory for safety
C. Discuss the issue privately with parents
D. Ignore the concern to avoid confrontation

Q554. A 6-year-old hospitalized for chemotherapy cries whenever the nurse enters the room. The most appropriate nursing action is to:
A. Limit visits to reduce anxiety
B. Allow the child to participate in care decisions when possible
C. Ask parents to stay away during procedures
D. Explain procedures in detail before each one

Q555. A 9-year-old child expresses fear that classmates will not accept them after hair loss from chemotherapy. The best nursing response is to:
A. Reassure that true friends will not care about appearance
B. Offer to arrange a peer education session at school
C. Suggest wearing a wig until hair regrows
D. Tell the child to avoid talking about it

Q556. A teenager with recurrent leukemia says, "I'm tired of fighting." The nurse's most appropriate response is to:
A. Encourage focusing on family and things that bring comfort
B. Tell the patient not to give up hope
C. Remind them of all the progress made so far
D. Ask if they want to talk about treatment options

Q557. The parents of a toddler newly diagnosed with lymphoma feel overwhelmed by complex discharge instructions. The nurse's priority action is to:
A. Provide written materials and schedule follow-up teaching
B. Encourage them to memorize essential steps immediately
C. Request that another staff member review the information
D. Reduce the amount of information shared
Q558. A nurse caring for a child undergoing a bone marrow transplant observes the sibling crying and saying, "I wish it wasn't me who had to donate." The best nursing response is to:
A. Ask parents to discuss it with the child later
B. Reassure that donating is a good thing to do
C. Validate the sibling's feelings and provide emotional support
D. Tell the sibling it will help save their brother's life
Q559. A 15-year-old expresses anger toward parents for "making all the decisions" about treatment. The nurse's best action is to:
A. Include the adolescent in care planning discussions
B. Remind them that parents are responsible for care
C. Defer discussions to the physician
D. Suggest journaling feelings privately
Q560. A 10-year-old recovering from leukemia treatment exhibits new onset of anxiety and refuses school attendance. The nurse should:
A. Collaborate with school staff to create a gradual reentry plan
B. Advise the family to force the child to attend
C. Explain that anxiety will resolve with time
D. Recommend complete homeschooling
Q561. During a family meeting, a nurse observes parents arguing about continuing aggressive treatment. The best immediate action is to:
A. Allow the physician to mediate later
B. End the meeting and reschedule
C. Redirect the conversation to medical details
D. Facilitate open discussion focusing on shared goals for the child
Q562. A child nearing end of life says, "I'm scared to sleep because I might not wake up." The nurse's best reply is to:
A. Sit with the child and ask about their fears
B. Reassure that sleep is safe and normal
C. Suggest relaxation techniques
D. Ask parents to provide comfort instead
Q563. A family expresses difficulty talking about their child's prognosis due to cultural beliefs about discussing death. The nurse's best action is to:
A. Ask how their beliefs can be respected while planning care
B. Explain the importance of open communication
C. Involve the hospital chaplain to mediate
D. Provide written information on palliative care
Q564. A parent expresses worry about explaining a sibling's death to the surviving 5-year-old. The nurse should recommend:
A. Describing death as "sleeping"
B. Avoiding the topic until the child asks questions
C. Using simple, concrete language that the child can understand
D. Allowing another relative to explain later
Q565. An adolescent patient reports feeling isolated because peers "don't understand cancer." The most effective nursing intervention is to:
A. Connect the patient with an adolescent cancer support group
B. Offer books about adolescent coping
C. Schedule family sessions instead
D. Encourage more visits from relatives
Q566. A single parent caring for a child with sickle cell disease expresses financial stress and fear of job loss. The nurse's best action is to:
A. Refer to a hospital social worker for resource assistance
B. Provide reassurance that things will work out
C. Offer personal coping suggestions
D. Focus discussion on treatment adherence
Q567. The nurse observes that a teenager with bone sarcoma withdrawing from friends after an amputation. The most therapeutic intervention is to:

A. Encourage participation in body image and peer support programs
B. Suggest spending more time with family
C. Focus only on physical rehabilitation progress
D. Recommend reading about others with disabilities

Q568. The parents of a terminally ill child say they no longer pray because "nothing changes." The nurse's best response is to:
A. Redirect the conversation to the care plan
B. Offer to pray with them immediately
C. Suggest talking to the chaplain without further discussion
D. Acknowledge their spiritual distress and explore what brings them comfort now

Q569. During teaching, a nurse notes that a caregiver repeatedly interrupts and expresses anger about the diagnosis. The most appropriate action is to:
A. Pause the session and explore the caregiver's emotional readiness
B. Continue teaching to cover all information
C. Ask another nurse to complete the session
D. Focus only on medical facts

Q570. A 6-year-old in remission from leukemia exhibits nightmares and separation anxiety when returning to school. The nurse's best intervention is to:
A. Encourage gradual exposure with support from teachers and parents
B. Reassure the child that dreams are not real
C. Recommend psychiatric medication evaluation
D. Limit discussions about cancer experiences

Q571. A nurse notices that a mother constantly checks on her hospitalized child and avoids leaving the room. The best initial nursing response is to:
A. Encourage the mother to rest outside occasionally
B. Explore her fears and provide reassurance about care
C. Limit visitation time to promote independence
D. Arrange counseling for anxiety management

Q572. A 12-year-old with leukemia feels guilty about causing family stress. The most therapeutic nurse response is to:
A. Clarify that illness is not anyone's fault
B. Divert the topic to something more positive
C. Ask the parents to reassure the child later
D. Explain that treatment will ease family burden

Q573. The parents of a child in palliative care argue about whether to continue aggressive treatment. The nurse's best action is to:
A. Facilitate a care conference to help them make unified decisions
B. Offer the physician's opinion for guidance
C. Encourage one parent to take the lead
D. Defer discussions until emotions settle

Q574. During a routine visit, a nurse observes a father of a child with sickle cell disease showing signs of withdrawal and irritability. The best nursing action is to:
A. Recommend rest breaks during hospitalization
B. Redirect focus to the child's progress
C. Assess for signs of caregiver burnout and offer support
D. Provide reading material about the disease

Q575. A 10-year-old patient asks, "Why do my parents cry every time the doctor talks to them?" The most appropriate nurse response is to:
A. Ask what the child thinks about their parents' reactions
B. Tell the child their parents are just tired
C. Avoid the question to prevent emotional distress
D. Suggest talking to the parents directly

Q576. A family from a non-English-speaking background seems confused during discharge teaching. The nurse should first:
A. Arrange for a professional medical interpreter
B. Simplify instructions and repeat them
C. Ask the child to translate for parents
D. Provide printed material in English

Q577. A nurse observes that a school-age child receiving long-term chemotherapy has become withdrawn and no longer enjoys playtime. The best intervention is to:
A. Inform parents to arrange counseling
B. Engage the child in therapeutic play to assess emotional state
C. Increase medication education sessions
D. Encourage more family visits

Q578. During a home visit, a nurse finds that parents of a child with hemophilia are hesitant to allow the child to play outside. The nurse's best teaching point is to:

A. Discuss safe activity options appropriate for the child's condition

B. Encourage complete restriction to prevent injuries

C. Recommend increased supervision during outdoor play

D. Suggest consulting the physician for clearance

Q579. The nurse observes that a sibling of a child with cancer begins acting out in school. The best nursing intervention is to:

A. Include the sibling in age-appropriate hospital activities

B. Focus on discipline strategies with parents

C. Provide written information about sibling reactions

D. Suggest reducing the sibling's school workload

Q580. A mother of a terminally ill child says, "I can't cry in front of my son; I have to be strong." The nurse's best response is to:

A. Suggest speaking with a counselor about grief later

B. Encourage the mother to cry privately only

C. Tell her it's important to hide emotions to avoid upsetting the child

D. Explain that sharing emotions models healthy coping for the child

Q581. An adolescent recently diagnosed with lymphoma refuses to attend a support group, saying, "I'm not like those kids." The nurse's best response is to:

A. Acknowledge the concern and explore personal preferences for support

B. Emphasize the value of meeting peers

C. Tell the patient to try it once before deciding

D. Ask parents to encourage participation

Q582. During rounds, a nurse finds a mother praying quietly and crying beside her child's bed. The most therapeutic action is to:

A. Sit quietly and offer presence without interruption

B. Ask if she would like the chaplain to visit

C. Leave to provide privacy

D. Remind her of upcoming medical rounds

Q583. A child receiving palliative chemotherapy tells the nurse, "I wish I could just go home." The best nursing response is to:

A. Change the topic to a lighter subject

B. Promise that discharge will happen soon

C. Explore what "home" means to the child and their wishes

D. Tell the parents privately about the request

Q584. A caregiver expresses feeling inadequate in administering home injections for a child with thalassemia. The nurse's best approach is to:

A. Demonstrate the technique again and offer supervised practice

B. Suggest that another family member take over

C. Reassure that fear is normal but not necessary

D. Provide a written guide without demonstration

Q585. A 13-year-old receiving radiation asks, "Will I ever be able to have children?" The nurse's most appropriate response is to:

A. Provide honest, age-appropriate information and offer to discuss fertility preservation

B. Defer discussion to the oncologist

C. Say the treatment won't affect fertility

D. Avoid answering to reduce distress

Q586. The nurse observes that grandparents caring for a child with chronic anemia seem overwhelmed and forget care instructions. The best nursing response is to:

A. Simplify teaching and use return demonstrations

B. Provide all education materials at once

C. Recommend transferring care to the parents

D. Focus only on written instructions

Q587. A teenager with a terminal diagnosis refuses to talk to anyone, saying, "What's the point?" The nurse's most effective approach is to:

A. Encourage focusing on enjoyable activities

B. Sit quietly and offer presence until the patient is ready to talk

C. Ask parents to stay and provide distraction

D. Change the subject to reduce discomfort

Q588. A parent insists that traditional healing rituals be performed before a child's transfusion. The nurse should:

A. Collaborate to safely accommodate the ritual within care parameters
B. Explain that hospital policies prohibit rituals
C. Ask the physician for permission first
D. Delay the ritual until discharge

Q589. A 6-year-old expresses sadness that "nobody wants to play" after returning from treatment. The nurse's best intervention is to:
A. Arrange a supervised playdate or peer reintegration activity
B. Advise parents to focus on academics instead
C. Recommend online games for distraction
D. Tell the child not to worry about friends

Q590. A nurse finds parents arguing over blame for their child's diagnosis. The most effective response is to:
A. Reassure that arguments are normal in crises
B. Ask them to discuss feelings privately
C. Address the emotional conflict and redirect focus toward coping together
D. Leave the room to allow privacy

Q591. A nurse caring for a child with relapsed leukemia notices that the parents speak only about medical treatments and avoid discussing emotions. The most appropriate nursing action is to:
A. Gently explore how the parents are coping emotionally
B. Focus strictly on treatment adherence to maintain professionalism
C. Wait for the parents to initiate discussion about feelings
D. Directly tell them to see a counselor

Q592. A 15-year-old patient expresses anger at God for "letting this happen." The nurse's best response is to:
A. Encourage the patient to share more about these feelings
B. Suggest that faith will eventually be restored
C. Avoid discussing religion to maintain boundaries
D. Tell the chaplain to visit without further discussion

Q593. A mother of a 5-year-old with sickle cell disease blames herself for passing on the condition. The most therapeutic nursing response is to:
A. Ask if she wants to meet other parents with the same diagnosis
B. Encourage her to focus on her child's progress
C. Redirect her toward treatment goals
D. Reassure that the disease is genetically inherited and not her fault

Q594. During a group session, an adolescent undergoing bone marrow transplant says, "I don't recognize myself anymore." The nurse's most effective intervention is to:
A. Encourage creative expression, such as journaling or art therapy
B. Remind the patient recovery will restore appearance
C. Suggest focusing on physical rehabilitation only
D. Avoid the topic to prevent distress

Q595. A 9-year-old patient undergoing chemotherapy is anxious before each treatment. The nurse's best initial action is to:
A. Offer age-appropriate teaching and relaxation techniques
B. Encourage parents to distract the child with toys
C. Administer sedatives before each session
D. Schedule treatments during quiet hours

Q596. A nurse notices that a father caring for a child with hemophilia refuses assistance from support groups. The nurse should:
A. Insist on participation in family support meetings
B. Respect his choice and periodically reassess readiness
C. Ask the social worker to persuade him
D. Avoid discussing the topic further

Q597. A family requests that the nurse not disclose a terminal prognosis to their 10-year-old child. The nurse's best action is to:
A. Discuss the family's reasons and collaborate on an age-appropriate communication plan
B. Respect the request and avoid the subject
C. Inform the child privately about their condition
D. Defer the issue entirely to the physician

Q598. A sibling of a hospitalized child says, "Everyone only cares about my sister now." The nurse's best response is to:

A. Acknowledge the feeling and offer attention through inclusion in care
B. Tell the sibling that their parents love them equally
C. Advise the parents to arrange more time together
D. Change the subject to something fun

Q599. During a home visit, a nurse observes that a child with chronic cancer pain spends most of the day alone in their room. The most therapeutic nursing action is to:

A. Limit family discussion about the illness
B. Respect the child's desire for privacy
C. Suggest referral to inpatient care
D. Encourage family interaction and structured daily routines

Q600. The parents of a terminally ill child express uncertainty about how to explain death to their younger children. The nurse's best recommendation is to:

A. Use clear, age-appropriate language and allow questions
B. Avoid discussing the topic until children ask
C. Describe death as "sleeping" to reduce fear
D. Ask a counselor to explain for them

Answer Key and Explanation (501-600)

Q501. Answer: A

Explanation: Transfusion-associated reactions may cause acute respiratory distress. Stopping the transfusion and maintaining IV access with saline prevent further antigen exposure while treatment is initiated.

Subdomain: Hypersensitivity – Transfusion Reaction

Q502. Answer: B

Explanation: Hydration dilutes serum solutes and promotes renal clearance of uric acid and potassium, reducing tumor lysis risk. Early intervention prevents renal failure and electrolyte imbalance.

Subdomain: Metabolic – Tumor Lysis Syndrome

Q503. Answer: A

Explanation: Prolonged priapism is a vaso-occlusive emergency. Hydration and analgesia reduce ischemia while preparing for possible aspiration by urology. Early intervention prevents tissue damage.

Subdomain: Vascular – Priapism

Q504. Answer: A

Explanation: Cytokine release syndrome triggers a massive inflammatory response that may lead to shock. Tocilizumab, an IL-6 inhibitor, mitigates the inflammatory cascade and stabilizes the patient.

Subdomain: Metabolic – Cytokine Release Syndrome

Q505. Answer: C

Explanation: Vaso-occlusive crisis causes ischemic pain from sickled cells obstructing blood flow. Hydration and opioid therapy relieve symptoms and improve circulation. Heat and rest may further support recovery.

Subdomain: Vascular – Vaso-occlusive Crisis

Q506. Answer: A

Explanation: When hypotension does not respond to fluids, septic shock is likely, and vasopressors are required to maintain perfusion. Continuous monitoring and antibiotic therapy are essential.

Subdomain: Infection – Septic Shock

Q507. Answer: A

Explanation: Vincristine-induced peripheral neuropathy can become irreversible. Prompt reporting allows for dosage modification or therapy change. Ongoing assessment prevents further neurological impairment.

Subdomain: Neurology – Drug-Induced Neuropathy

Q508. Answer: D

Explanation: Donor immune cells attacking host tissues cause graft-versus-host disease, commonly affecting skin, liver, and GI tract. Immunosuppressive therapy must be initiated immediately.

Subdomain: Immune – Graft-versus-Host Disease

Q509. Answer: A

Explanation: Anthracycline drugs like daunorubicin can cause cardiotoxicity, reflected by reduced ejection fraction. Cardiac monitoring detects early myocardial damage, allowing therapy modification.

Subdomain: Cardiopulmonary – Cardiotoxicity

Q510. Answer: A

Explanation: Hyponatremia due to SIADH causes neurologic symptoms from cerebral edema. Controlled fluid restriction and hypertonic saline correct sodium safely. Continuous neurologic monitoring is critical.

Subdomain: Metabolic – SIADH

Q511. Answer: B

Explanation: Tumor lysis syndrome causes electrolyte disturbances from rapid tumor cell destruction. Elevated phosphorus binds calcium, resulting in hypocalcemia and neuromuscular irritability. Aggressive hydration and monitoring are vital.

Subdomain: Metabolic – Tumor Lysis Syndrome

Q512. Answer: B

Explanation: Ifosfamide encephalopathy results from neurotoxic metabolites. Methylene blue reverses this process by improving mitochondrial function. The drug should be stopped immediately and neuro checks continued.

Subdomain: Neurology – Drug-Induced Encephalopathy

Q513. Answer: A

Explanation: Sinusoidal obstructive syndrome presents with hepatic congestion after transplant conditioning. Defibrotide improves microcirculation and decreases mortality. Early detection prevents liver failure.

Subdomain: Vascular – Sinusoidal Obstructive Syndrome

Q514. Answer: A

Explanation: Vaso-occlusive crisis results from impaired blood flow due to sickled cells. Hydration and opioids relieve ischemic pain and restore perfusion. Rest and warmth support recovery.

Subdomain: Vascular – Vaso-occlusive Crisis

Q515. Answer: C

Explanation: Fever and hypotension during transfusion may signal sepsis or anaphylaxis. Immediate discontinuation of transfusion and saline maintenance prevent further antigen exposure while treatment begins.

Subdomain: Hypersensitivity – Transfusion Reaction

Q516. Answer: A

Explanation: Headache and vomiting without nausea are classic signs of increased intracranial pressure. Elevating the head of the bed and notifying the provider help prevent herni, herniation. Frequent neuro checks are essential.

Subdomain: Neurology – Increased Intracranial Pressure

Q517. Answer: A

Explanation: Cytokine release syndrome produces systemic inflammation and vascular leakage. Tocilizumab blocks IL-6, rapidly improving hemodynamics. Continuous vital-sign monitoring ensures early stabilization.

Subdomain: Metabolic – Cytokine Release Syndrome

Q518. Answer: D

Explanation: Immediate factor replacement halts bleeding and prevents hemarthrosis complications. Ice and immobilization follow to reduce swelling. Delayed replacement risks chronic joint damage.

Subdomain: Vascular – Joint Bleed (Hemophilia)

Q519. Answer: A

Explanation: Vincristine can cause peripheral neuropathy leading to motor deficits. Prompt reporting allows dose adjustment or drug substitution. Early detection prevents irreversible nerve injury.

Subdomain: Neurology – Drug-Induced Neuropathy

Q520. Answer: A

Explanation: These signs indicate superior vena cava syndrome from mediastinal compression. Elevating the head facilitates venous drainage and reduces pressure until medical treatment begins.

Subdomain: Cardiopulmonary – Superior Vena Cava Syndrome

Q521. Answer: C

Explanation: SIADH leads to water retention and dilutional hyponatremia, producing neurologic symptoms. Fluid restriction and sodium correction are critical to prevent seizures and cerebral edema.

Subdomain: Metabolic – SIADH

Q522. Answer: A

Explanation: Acute chest syndrome requires oxygenation to relieve hypoxia and antibiotics for infection control. Early intervention prevents respiratory failure and cardiac strain.

Subdomain: Cardiopulmonary – Acute Chest Syndrome

Q523. Answer: A

Explanation: Hemorrhagic cystitis results from bladder irritation by cyclophosphamide metabolites. Vigorous hydration flushes toxins, and mesna may be prescribed for protection. Prompt action prevents permanent injury.

Subdomain: Genitourinary – Hemorrhagic Cystitis

Q524. Answer: D

Explanation: Anthracycline cardiotoxicity reduces ejection fraction, detectable on echocardiogram. Regular cardiac monitoring identifies dysfunction early for dose adjustment or discontinuation.

Subdomain: Cardiopulmonary – Cardiotoxicity

Q525. Answer: A

Explanation: Pancreatitis is a serious asparaginase complication requiring immediate discontinuation. Supportive management with fasting and IV fluids prevents further pancreatic damage.

Subdomain: Gastrointestinal – Pancreatitis

Q526. Answer: A

Explanation: PRES presents with seizures and visual changes linked to immunosuppressant toxicity or hypertension. Control of blood pressure and adjustment of medication reverse symptoms.

Subdomain: Neurology – PRES

Q527. Answer: B

Explanation: Donor immune cells attacking host tissues cause graft-versus-host disease. Skin, liver, and GI involvement require prompt immunosuppressive treatment to prevent systemic damage.

Subdomain: Immune – Graft-versus-Host Disease

Q528. Answer: A

Explanation: Persistent hypotension despite fluids indicates septic shock requiring vasopressors such as dopamine or norepinephrine. Rapid intervention maintains tissue perfusion and oxygenation.

Subdomain: Infection – Septic Shock

Q529. Answer: A

Explanation: Priapism results from sickled-cell blockage in penile vasculature. Rapid urologic evaluation and exchange transfusion may be necessary to prevent ischemic injury.

Subdomain: Vascular – Priapism

Q530. Answer: D

Explanation: Methotrexate toxicity worsens in acidic urine. Maintaining alkalinized urine and providing leucovorin rescue prevent renal and CNS injury. Continuous monitoring of renal function is essential.

Subdomain: Metabolic – Drug-Induced Toxicity

Q531. Answer: B

Explanation: Adolescents with body image changes often need space to express grief and anger before accepting adaptation. Allowing open emotional expression helps restore trust and encourages eventual participation in therapy. This approach supports emotional adjustment and self-efficacy in rehabilitation.

Subdomain: Principles of growth and development

Q532. Answer: A

Explanation: Families often cycle through stages of grief following a child's diagnosis. Recognizing these emotional responses as normal reduces guilt and supports coping. The nurse validates their feelings and gradually guides them toward acceptance.

Subdomain: Social relationships and family dynamics

Q533. Answer: B

Explanation: Exploring the emotional meaning behind pain allows the nurse to identify underlying fear or depression. This strategy promotes emotional insight and builds trust. Addressing psychosocial distress is crucial in chronic illness care.

Subdomain: Mental health

Q534. Answer: A

Explanation: Family meetings help align communication and clarify goals of care in emotionally charged situations. Involving the interdisciplinary team ensures ethical, family-centered decision-making. This approach reduces conflict and promotes unity in care.

Subdomain: Family dynamics and support

Q535. Answer: B

Explanation: Honest yet age-appropriate communication supports trust and emotional safety. Acknowledging fears about pain and explaining comfort measures helps children cope with uncertainty. This fosters a sense of control and peace.

Subdomain: Grief and bereavement

Q536. Answer: B

Explanation: Misconceptions among peers can worsen social isolation. Coordinating with school personnel to provide accurate information reduces stigma and promotes reintegration. Advocacy supports the child's social and emotional well-being.

Subdomain: Community resources

Q537. Answer: A

Explanation: Parental guilt is common and can hinder coping. Reassuring parents that pediatric cancers are not caused by parental actions helps alleviate emotional distress. This creates a foundation for healthy adjustment.

Subdomain: Cultural considerations and diversity

Q538. Answer: A
Explanation: Adolescents need peer connection to maintain self-concept. Expressive writing and peer groups offer safe outlets for emotions and identity affirmation. These interventions promote resilience and belonging.
Subdomain: Psychosocial development
Q539. Answer: D
Explanation: Culturally competent care begins with understanding family beliefs before giving education or recommendations. Building respect fosters trust and adherence. Collaboration ensures safety while honoring cultural values.
Subdomain: Cultural considerations and diversity
Q540. Answer: A
Explanation: Emotional assessment is essential to holistic nursing care. Addressing distress early prevents caregiver burnout and supports effective home management. This promotes long-term family resilience.
Subdomain: Family support and education
Q541. Answer: A
Explanation: Expressions of hopelessness in serious illness may signal depression or suicidal thoughts. Early assessment enables timely mental health referral and safety planning. The nurse plays a key role in identifying risk.
Subdomain: Mental health
Q542. Answer: C
Explanation: Taste alterations are common during therapy and may affect family routines. Encouraging small, family-oriented meals promotes comfort and emotional support. Family involvement reinforces normalcy.
Subdomain: Growth and development principles
Q543. Answer: A
Explanation: Caregiver fatigue impacts both emotional and physical health. Connecting families with respite or community support prevents burnout and enhances care continuity. Empowering families strengthens coping capacity.
Subdomain: Community resources
Q544. Answer: A
Explanation: Supporting positive body image through choice and preparation promotes self-esteem. Encouraging autonomy helps children manage appearance changes confidently. This builds adaptive coping skills.
Subdomain: Growth and development principles
Q545. Answer: D
Explanation: Compassionate follow-up extends continuity of care into the bereavement phase. Providing resources and emotional support assists families in healthy mourning. This reflects holistic, family-centered care.
Subdomain: Grief and bereavement
Q546. Answer: A
Explanation: Joint participation promotes shared responsibility and reduces conflict. Collaborative education fosters teamwork and confidence in caregiving. This supports safety and strengthens family unity.
Subdomain: Family dynamics and support
Q547. Answer: A
Explanation: Supporting autonomy and peer engagement helps maintain identity and emotional health. Encouraging alternative social outlets meets developmental needs while respecting limitations. This fosters resilience.
Subdomain: Psychosocial development
Q548. Answer: C
Explanation: Involving siblings reduces jealousy and fosters understanding of the ill child's condition. Age-appropriate inclusion maintains family cohesion. This promotes emotional balance within the family unit.
Subdomain: Family dynamics and support
Q549. Answer: A
Explanation: Parental presence enhances security and cooperation in young children. Allowing involvement reduces fear and supports trust. This approach respects developmental and emotional needs.
Subdomain: Growth and development principles
Q550. Answer: A
Explanation: Validating conflicting emotions helps parents process anticipatory grief without shame. Recognizing such feelings as part of compassionate love eases guilt. This nurtures acceptance and emotional healing.
Subdomain: Grief and bereavement
Q551. Answer: B
Explanation: Honest, developmentally appropriate discussion fosters trust and helps

children process fears realistically. Inviting the child to express understanding encourages open communication. This approach reduces anxiety and promotes coping.
Subdomain: Principles of growth and development

Q552. Answer: B

Explanation: Emotional exhaustion from repeated hospitalizations is common. Acknowledging feelings and connecting families to community or respite resources strengthens coping and resilience. Compassionate listening promotes trust and engagement in care.
Subdomain: Community resources

Q553. Answer: A

Explanation: Adolescents seek independence and individuality. Supporting self-expression while maintaining safety encourages compliance without compromising identity. This strategy enhances collaboration and self-care confidence.
Subdomain: Psychosocial development

Q554. Answer: B

Explanation: Allowing control within safe limits gives children a sense of autonomy and security. Involving them in small choices reduces fear and builds trust. Empowerment is key to reducing procedural anxiety.
Subdomain: Growth and development principles

Q555. Answer: B

Explanation: Facilitating education for peers promotes understanding and reduces social stigma. Proactive communication helps the child feel supported and fosters reintegration. This strengthens self-esteem and belonging.
Subdomain: Community resources

Q556. Answer: A

Explanation: Acknowledging emotional fatigue respects the patient's experience without forcing optimism. Encouraging focus on comfort and meaning fosters emotional peace. This aligns with palliative and psychosocial care principles.
Subdomain: Grief and bereavement

Q557. Answer: A

Explanation: Providing written instructions and repetition supports adult learning and retention under stress. Spaced teaching ensures safe and confident home care. Effective communication reduces anxiety and errors.
Subdomain: Family education and support

Q558. Answer: C

Explanation: Donor siblings may experience guilt, fear, or resentment. Validating emotions helps normalize these feelings and prevents long-term distress. Emotional support fosters psychological safety and family harmony.
Subdomain: Family dynamics and support

Q559. Answer: A

Explanation: Adolescents need autonomy and involvement to foster trust and compliance. Including them in decisions respects developmental needs and promotes collaboration. This enhances emotional adjustment to illness.
Subdomain: Growth and development principles

Q560. Answer: A

Explanation: Gradual reentry programs supported by teachers and healthcare teams help children regain confidence and social
social stability. Coordination reduces fear and promotes reintegration. This supports long-term psychosocial recovery.
Subdomain: Community resources

Q561. Answer: D

Explanation: Encouraging shared dialogue promotes mutual understanding and unified decision-making. The nurse's role as a facilitator ensures emotional expression within a structured, compassionate setting. This maintains family cohesion and focus on the child's well-being.
Subdomain: Family dynamics and support

Q562. Answer: A

Explanation: Offering presence and inviting expression of fear provides emotional safety. Active listening allows the child to articulate concerns and regain control. This response demonstrates compassionate, child-centered communication.
Subdomain: Grief and bereavement

Q563. Answer: A

Explanation: Exploring cultural perspectives demonstrates respect and supports individualized care. Understanding beliefs allows nurses to align communication styles

appropriately. This builds trust and promotes culturally sensitive care.
Subdomain: Cultural considerations and diversity
Q564. Answer: C
Explanation: Young children interpret information literally; clear, simple explanations prevent confusion and fear. Honest communication fosters healthy grieving. This supports normal developmental processing of loss.
Subdomain: Grief and bereavement
Q565. Answer: A
Explanation: Peer support groups provide normalization and shared understanding of illness experiences. These interactions fulfill developmental needs for social connection and identity. Such peer relationships enhance emotional well-being.
Subdomain: Psychosocial development
Q566. Answer: A
Explanation: Addressing socioeconomic challenges ensures comprehensive, family-centered care. Connecting parents with social work resources reduces stress and improves treatment compliance. Interdisciplinary collaboration enhances stability.
Subdomain: Socioeconomic issues
Q567. Answer: A
Explanation: Addressing altered body image through support programs promotes confidence and peer reintegration. Emotional acceptance improves quality of life and self-esteem. Holistic support fosters adjustment.
Subdomain: Psychosocial development
Q568. Answer: D
Explanation: Recognizing spiritual distress validates complex emotions during grief. Exploring sources of comfort promotes healing and helps families redefine meaning. This supports holistic, compassionate care.
Subdomain: Cultural considerations and diversity
Q569. Answer: A
Explanation: Emotional readiness affects comprehension and coping. Pausing to assess feelings allows the nurse to address distress before resuming education. This patient-centered approach enhances learning and trust.
Subdomain: Family education and support
Q570. Answer: A
Explanation: Gradual reintroduction with consistent support helps children regain confidence after trauma. Collaboration between family and school normalizes the transition. This promotes emotional recovery and adaptation.
Subdomain: Principles of growth and development
Q571. Answer: B
Explanation: Parental hypervigilance often stems from fear of losing control or distrust in care. Exploring the mother's worries and offering reassurance builds confidence in the healthcare team. This supports a therapeutic partnership and reduces anxiety.
Subdomain: Family dynamics and support
Q572. Answer: A
Explanation: Guilt is a common emotional reaction among ill children. Clarifying that illness is not self-caused relieves emotional distress and fosters self-worth. Honest reassurance strengthens coping and emotional recovery.
Subdomain: Mental health
Q573. Answer: A
Explanation: A structured family meeting promotes shared understanding and aligns goals of care. Facilitating communication with the interdisciplinary team ensures ethical and compassionate decisions. This reduces conflict and emotional strain.
Subdomain: Family dynamics and support
Q574. Answer: C
Explanation: Caregiver burnout can lead to emotional exhaustion and poor family functioning. Early assessment and support prevent deterioration of mental health. Providing coping resources promotes sustainable caregiving.
Subdomain: Family education and support
Q575. Answer: A
Explanation: Inviting the child to share perceptions allows expression of fears and misconceptions. It provides insight into emotional needs while maintaining honesty. This

supports developmentally appropriate communication.
Subdomain: Growth and development principles
Q576. Answer: A
Explanation: Using certified interpreters ensures accuracy and cultural sensitivity in communication. This approach prevents misunderstanding and promotes safe, equitable care. Cultural competence is essential in pediatric oncology nursing.
Subdomain: Cultural considerations and diversity
Q577. Answer: B
Explanation: Therapeutic play offers a safe medium for children to express emotions they may not verbalize. It allows nurses to identify anxiety or depression early. This strategy enhances coping and emotional adjustment.
Subdomain: Psychosocial development
Q578. Answer: A
Explanation: Overprotection can limit social and emotional growth. Teaching families about safe activities balances protection with developmental needs. Promoting age-appropriate independence fosters confidence and well-being.
Subdomain: Growth and development principles
Q579. Answer: A
Explanation: Sibling acting out often reflects unmet emotional needs or jealousy. Inclusion in care promotes understanding and reduces feelings of neglect. This approach supports healthy family adjustment.
Subdomain: Family dynamics and support
Q580. Answer: D
Explanation: Open emotional expression normalizes grief for children and fosters honest communication. It helps the child process emotions safely. Modeling vulnerability teaches acceptance of difficult feelings.
Subdomain: Grief and bereavement
Q581. Answer: A
Explanation: Respecting individuality allows the adolescent to maintain autonomy. Exploring alternative support forms encourages emotional openness without pressure. This builds trust and engagement.
Subdomain: Psychosocial development
Q582. Answer: A
Explanation: Silent presence conveys empathy and support during spiritual distress. Nonverbal compassion often provides greater comfort than words. This fosters trust and emotional relief.
Subdomain: Cultural considerations and diversity
Q583. Answer: C
Explanation: Exploring the child's statement provides insight into emotional needs and end-of-life concerns. Understanding meaning promotes patient-centered communication. This ensures compassionate and individualized care.
Subdomain: Grief and bereavement
Q584. Answer: A
Explanation: Reinforcing psychomotor skills through hands-on demonstration enhances confidence and competence. Addressing emotional barriers directly encourages success. This approach supports family empowerment and safe care.
Subdomain: Family education and support
Q585. Answer: A
Explanation: Adolescents are capable of understanding reproductive health implications. Honest communication and early counseling promote informed choices and trust. This reflects respect for developing autonomy.
Subdomain: Growth and development principles
Q586. Answer: A
Explanation: Adapting teaching methods to caregiver ability ensures understanding and safety. Combining demonstration with repetition supports retention and confidence. This promotes consistent, quality home care.
Subdomain: Family education and support
Q587. Answer: B
Explanation: Silence and presence communicate respect and emotional availability. Allowing space fosters trust and facilitates later expression of grief. This compassionate approach supports dignity and connection.
Subdomain: Grief and bereavement
Q588. Answer: A
Explanation: Integrating safe cultural practices enhances family comfort and trust. Collaboration respects belief systems while

maintaining medical safety. This supports culturally competent, family-centered care.
Subdomain: Cultural considerations and diversity

Q589. Answer: A

Explanation: Social reintegration supports emotional recovery and developmental progress. Encouraging safe peer interactions rebuilds confidence and normalcy. Play is a critical medium for pediatric adaptation.
Subdomain: Psychosocial development

Q590. Answer: C

Explanation: Addressing guilt and blame directly helps families move toward mutual support. Guided communication restores collaboration and reduces emotional strain. The nurse facilitates unity during stressful times.
Subdomain: Family dynamics and support

Q591. Answer: A

Explanation: Families facing relapse often suppress emotions as a coping mechanism. Exploring their feelings with sensitivity helps identify hidden distress and promotes healthy expression. Emotional validation is key to long-term coping.
Subdomain: Family dynamics and support

Q592. Answer: A

Explanation: Spiritual anger is a normal aspect of adolescent coping during illness. Encouraging dialogue allows the nurse to support exploration and healing. Open listening facilitates spiritual resilience.
Subdomain: Cultural considerations and diversity

Q593. Answer: D

Explanation: Guilt from genetic transmission is a common emotional reaction. Providing factual reassurance alleviates misplaced blame and fosters emotional relief. This enhances parental confidence and bonding.
Subdomain: Mental health

Q594. Answer: A

Explanation: Identity disruption is common in adolescents facing altered body image. Creative expression provides safe outlets for self-reflection and emotional healing. This fosters acceptance and self-confidence.
Subdomain: Psychosocial development

Q595. Answer: A

Explanation: Understanding and predictability reduce procedural anxiety in children. Combining education with coping techniques empowers the child and promotes trust. This strengthens resilience and cooperation.
Subdomain: Growth and development principles

Q596. Answer: B

Explanation: Readiness to accept help varies among caregivers. Respecting autonomy while maintaining open communication preserves trust. Ongoing assessment ensures timely support when needed.
Subdomain: Family education and support

Q597. Answer: A

Explanation: Balancing honesty with cultural and family values is crucial in pediatric communication. Collaboration preserves trust and ethical integrity. This approach supports family unity while safeguarding the child's emotional needs.
Subdomain: Cultural considerations and diversity

Q598. Answer: A

Explanation: Siblings often experience jealousy or neglect during prolonged illness. Inclusion and acknowledgment validate their emotions and restore balance. This intervention supports family harmony and coping.
Subdomain: Family dynamics and support

Q599. Answer: D

Explanation: Isolation increases risk for depression and family detachment. Encouraging shared activities restores connection and emotional stability. Structured support enhances overall quality of life.
Subdomain: Mental health

Q600. Answer: A

Explanation: Honest, simple explanations help children process loss realistically. Allowing questions supports emotional understanding and prevents confusion. This approach fosters healthy family communication during bereavement.
Subdomain: Grief and bereavement

Made in United States
Orlando, FL
05 November 2026

90229885R00081